It's All in the Record

Meeting the Challenge of Open Recording

Liz O'Rourke and Hazel Grant

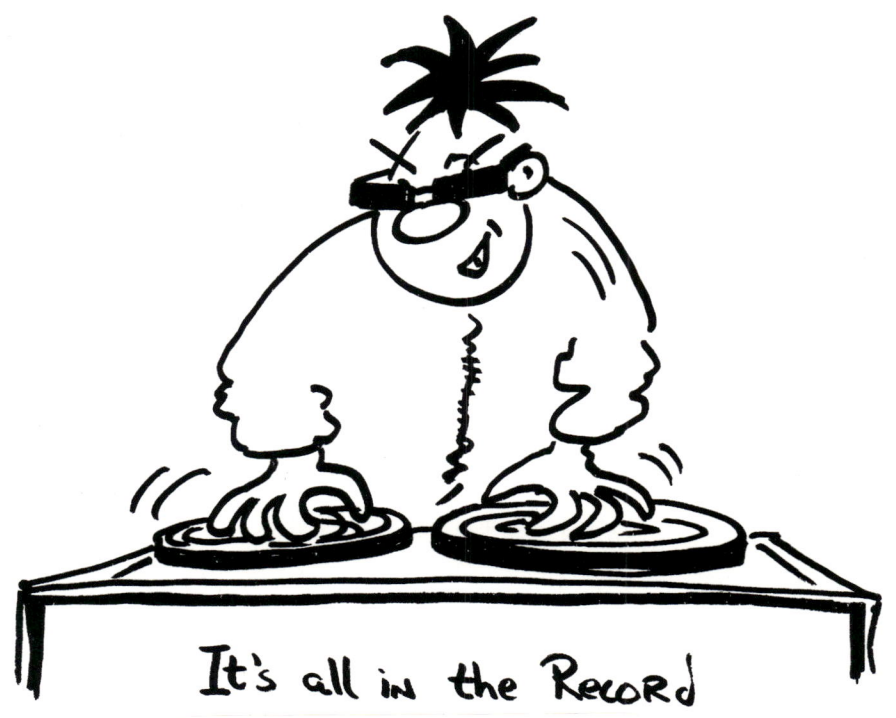

It's all in the Record

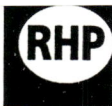

Russell House Publishing

First published in 2005 by:
Russell House Publishing Ltd.
4 St George's House
Uplyme Road
Lyme Regis
Dorset DT7 3LS

Tel: 01297-443948
Fax: 01297-442722
e-mail: help@russellhouse.co.uk
www.russellhouse.co.uk

British Library Cataloguing-in-publication Data:
A catalogue record for this book is available from the British Library.

ISBN: 1-903855-72-1

Typeset by TW Typesetting, Plymouth, Devon

Printed by Antony Rowe, Chippenham

Russell House Publishing

Is a group of social work, probation, education and youth and
community work practitioners and academics working in collaboration
with a professional publishing team.
Our aim is to work closely with the field to produce innovative and
valuable materials to help managers, trainers, practitioners
and students.
We are keen to receive feedback on publications and new ideas for
future projects.

Contents

Preface

Since writing *For the Record*, aimed mainly at direct care workers, I have been working more closely with care managers and social workers, exploring why so many practitioners struggle with case recording. One of the most significant challenges they encounter is that much of their recording is in the form of assessments, which are shared with a range of readerships, including service users. Many workers have described the dilemma of trying to record meaningful information about a service user and their situation without causing them discomfort or embarrassment. I have also worked with domiciliary carers, who are now expected to make records which are kept in the service user's home. Both of these groups of workers struggle with curiously similar issues.

This second manual explores the problems experienced by both care managers and home care workers in reconciling the tensions within open recording. My experience has been mainly with those employed in adult services, and so the case material in this manual has been developed in response to trying to meet their learning needs.

I am writing this manual with a co-author, Hazel Grant, who has extensive experience in working with issues around data protection and how information is used and shared by social services. We have each taken the lead responsibility for different sections of the manual, in line with our respective areas of expertise. The Introduction, Chapters 1, 2, 3, and 5 have been written by myself and Chapter 4 has been written by Hazel.

About the Authors

Liz O'Rourke is a training consultant (Tel.: 01865 741615), was previously a training manager with Berkshire Social Services, and has had wide experience in care work.

Hazel Grant has 18 years' experience in social work in London, Kent and Warwickshire, and is currently responsible for providing strategic information systems training, and Data Protection/Freedom of Information advice, in Warwickshire Social Services.

Acknowledgements

We are grateful to the various people who have provided encouragement in the writing of this manual. In particular we would like to thank, from Warwickshire Social Services: Ann Morrison, Assistant Service Manager, Disability Services, for her many helpful comments and suggestions on the draft manual; and Diana King, Team Manager, Health, for her contribution to the assessment objectives section in Chapter 2.

The manual has arisen out of the work undertaken with many learners and it is to them we owe a special thanks. Their contributions and participation during different training programmes have helped develop the ideas and approaches taken in this manual.

Last but in no way least, we'd like to thank our respective partners, Michael Clarke and John Grant for their support and forbearance while work has been in progress.

About the Cartoons and the Cartoonist

As often happens when cartoons are included in textbooks, practice guides and training manuals the ones in this book have already generated lively discussion.

During this discussion, someone asked the publisher to ask the cartoonist, Dug, why no black people appear in the cartoons. His response, which follows immediately here includes:

- information about the cartoonist
- thoughts on producing and publishing cartoons
- views on diversity in cartoons

A number of people have already commented that these views are interesting in their own right, and they have therefore been included in this book. If anyone would like to participate in a continuation of this debate with the cartoonist, or correspond with him for any other reason, he can be contacted on douglas@racionzer.net

On cartoons

Most of my colleagues find the question 'why no black people appear in the cartoons' incomprehensible. I live in South Africa, where we are struggling to reconcile with each other and build a nation with forgiveness and justice at its heart. We have many deep and intractable problems with which our racist past has left us. In our organisation we work in over 25 townships developing small and micro-enterprises. Every day we deal with the poison that Apartheid fed our people. This poison is that we believe we are second-rate, throwaway people, conquered, enslaved and colonised people. As part of our programme, I run cartooning workshops with children and adults, with corporate managers and artists and we engage the problems and opportunities that cartooning presents us.

I don't believe that cartooning is an art form but rather a broad approach to drawing that allows both drawer and reader the opportunity to recognize themselves in a fantasy world, a world of inordinate possibilities where the usual rules of daily life may be suspended and reworked to our advantage and often with humour. Cartoons allow us to see ourselves in the figures and situations drawn as impossibly simple and impossibly other. Cartoons give the child in all of us the chance to be and do anything that can be drawn.

How we see cartoons

If you don't see any black people in my cartoons, that's your perception. The cartoonist relies in large measure on the reader's common-sense stocks of knowledge to make the cartoons understood. If the reader sees no black people then I have failed to access the reader's sense of what black people look like in a cartoon.

All of us, including readers of cartoons maintain a memory of what various sorts of people look like. This stored memory contains templates of fat, thin, black, Indian, disabled, old, young and white people.

Visual media can be used for many purposes and these purposes in turn dictate the forms and subject matter.

The cartoons I draw in this book are imbedded in the text. The cartoons serve the author's intention of gaining the attention of the reader and ensuring the reader retains the meaning contained in the narrative. Placing a cartoon next to a heading in this book offers the reader the opportunity to integrate the meaning of a section of the book using parts of themselves that are not strictly intellectual but that may resonate at an emotional, subconscious level within the reader. Humour helps the reader to absorb the content, even perhaps by-passing the more consciously constructed and maintained perceptual filters we use when reading words.

Issues of technique

There are at least six gambits that cartoonists use to draw black people. Each strategy is in some way flawed and unsatisfactory.

1. Using colour may be the best way out but there is a limited budget and colour printing is still very expensive. In addition, the cartoons are designed to assist and support the text, not upstage the text. A colour cartoon may well overwhelm the heading and thus the whole point of drawing the cartoon to reinforce the meaning of the text will be lost.
2. Using racialised features such as crissy hair, thick lips and a squashed flat nose would simply be reinforcing untrue and silly racial stereotypes.
3. Using shading in black line drawings on white paper generally denotes texture and grittiness to the surface. It perhaps still needs to be said that black people do not have rougher, grittier skins than whites.
4. Using anthropomorphic figures is not funny to me and I hate drawing animals.
5. Using accessories can be just as stereotyping as drawing crude racial features. Not all people who have dreadlocks are pot smoking Rastas. Not all lesbians wear overalls with peace signs on them. Not all Indians wear turbans or fezzes.
6. Using a disclaimer to the effect that *'all the figures drawn in this cartoon do not represent any real person and are just the product of the cartoonist's fevered imagination'* would take up space and detract from the purpose of the cartoon, which is to support the narrative.

What is needed is something more profound, more ethically sound, more transformational than the usual cartooning techniques deployed presently. To this end I have crafted a set of stylistic pointers to drawing cartoons which may lead cartoonists and readers away from the mere replication of racial stereotypes.

A minimalist style

I have deliberately chosen a style that:

1. Is minimalist to the extent that there are not many details drawn.
2. The line drawings are androgynous, most of the figures could be male or female. I have stripped them of cues that engender or racialise them.
3. I have chosen to render figures and situations that reinforce the heading as much as possible and do not distract the reader from the text.
4. I only shade clothing to add more presence to the picture.
5. I have attempted to draw cartoons that are as transparent as possible so that the author's meaning can be impressed upon the reader without any other issues intervening or perceptual filters coming into play.

This stylistic strategy allows me to support the narrative and meaning of the book without relying on the cartoonist's usual shorthand in depicting gender or race. My skill is limited and I may fail to achieve these aims but it is nonetheless a deliberate and carefully chosen strategy on my part.

Cartoons and the real world

Unlike photography or caricature or portraiture, cartoons are not bound to a strictly representational rule for the subjects they draw but are more about situations than people. Animated cartoons are notorious for their displays of violence and all manner of criminal behaviour. Such behaviour is not acceptable in the real world and photographic depictions of real people doing these acts are rightfully deemed reprehensible. Our society however has no qualms with cartoonists drawing all sorts of vile and despicable acts of violence showing decapitations, murders and the like.

I doubt if any reader will complain about the cartoon in this book showing the person being run over by a bus and I have **not** been challenged about the levels of violence depicted in my cartoons. This failure to challenge me about my portrayal of violence is not really a failure but exposes a commonsense understanding we all share, that cartoons are not 'real, they do not depict the real life experiences of real people but they are understood to present an idea, a circumstance, a feeling. Our common-sense stocks of knowledge have a category for 'cartoons' and these cartoons are allowed great latitude in what the characters drawn do and say.

The real politics

I find representational politics and the notion that someone or something can represent me demeaning and sterile. I support the idea that we can only represent ourselves, that leaders are precisely that, leaders. Not 'representatives' of us or our interests. In like manner, my cartooning cannot claim to represent any live person or situation. The reader uses the images and words they read to construct in their mind's eye the meaning that they understand. The readers are responsible for 'seeing' what they see. This 'seeing' is a social action requiring detailed knowledge and skills. Perhaps placing this kind of seeing in perspective, allows me to introduce you to a more global perspective with regard to social action.

I am part of a fellowship that seeks to change this world and to build solutions to its problems using organisations and people who see themselves as global citizens. The Ashoka Fellowship is made up of about 1500 fellows in 53 countries worldwide.

Let me introduce you to some of our number:

- Nicole Rycroft from Canada runs Markets Initiative and had by 2003 convinced 32 Canadian publishing houses to use Ancient forest-friendly book grade paper.
- Jose Campana from Uruguay runs Book Banks where children are taught to restore books and maintain school libraries.
- Magda Iskander from Cairo has established homebound elder care as a profession in Egypt.
- Duke Kaufman runs the Sanctuary using old mine hostels in South Africa. The Sanctuary is the largest Aids orphanage in the world.
- Socorro Guteres in Brazil runs the Centre for Black Culture of Maranhao.
- Krzysztof Cyzewski runs the Borderland Foundation in Poland and wants to document and publish the achievements of young people in the ethnically diverse region of Sejny.
- Kim Feinberg in South Africa runs the Foundation for Tolerance Education.
- Rajidt Malley from Indonesia runs YLL and works with Gerperindo to highlight the illegal logging of indigenous forests.
- The Ashoka Fellowship www.ashoka.org is building a network of social entrepreneurs who are concerned with education, public welfare and the environment. We Ashoka Fellows need your support, your social action, your empathy, we need you to work with us and in practical ways, empower and give dignity to racially and ethnically diverse peoples who are often exploited by large multinational companies and by those with wealth and power.

I hope that these thoughts and insights are interesting and helpful. If anyone would like to discuss them with me, please email me on douglas@racionzer.net

Introduction

Meeting the challenge of open recording

Since the introduction of Access to Records legislation in the late 1980s, both health and social services are aware that users of their services have a right to see their records. This has had a profound impact on practice, with far more care now taken over how information is recorded.

The Data Protection Act 1998 has also influenced the way agencies record and share information. Confidentiality has long been an area of concern. The Data Protection Act has concentrated people's attention on how those principles of confidentiality are applied practically in the day-to-day work of health and social care agencies. Information Governance, arising from the Caldicott Report (1997) into information handling in the NHS, came into social care agencies in 2001. It provides a comprehensive and ethical framework for handling and sharing the highly personal information that such agencies manage. The electronic social care record is now a requirement.

Practitioners are familiar with the need to work in a more open and inclusive way with service users. Care managers and social workers are required to share copies of their assessments with their service users. More attempts are being made by direct care staff to include service users in the recording process. Home care staff make records which are kept in service users' homes. These are positive developments in the way we record, encouraging a more person-centred approach. However, they do give rise to a number of dilemmas for practitioners. How do you make effective recordings which are going to communicate useful and necessary information to other colleagues and still maintain a good relationship with your service user? When things run smoothly, this can be fairly straightforward. There are occasions however, when real difficulties can arise. This manual attempts to explore these dilemmas and suggest ways to address them.

Who is the manual for?

The manual is mainly directed towards trainers and managers who are responsible for developing practice in recording skills amongst care managers in adult social services. It will also have increasing relevance for those health workers who become care co-ordinators, as single, shared and unified assessments are established.

Although the principal focus is on addressing the needs of care managers in relation to recording, there is a section which specifically explores the recording task faced by home care workers. They are included in this manual because of its focus on open recording.

How does this manual relate to *For the Record*?

There may be people who, having bought the first manual will be wondering whether there is any point in buying another one. Surely there can't be anything more to be said on the subject? In the same way, many participants who attend my training courses often comment on arrival that they didn't think there was much to be said on recording, and certainly not enough to fill a whole day, let alone two days. They invariably leave with a rather more positive perspective on recording. Managers and trainers sometimes also make overly generalised assumptions about how to develop recording practice. Recording skills training is a neglected area where the actual learning needs are often poorly understood.

Recording skills are usually seen as a general training need in social care, which applies to all groups of workers, direct care workers, social workers and occupational therapists. If there is any distinction made between them in terms of their learning needs in relation to recording, it is on the basis of their different qualifications, i.e. direct care workers have S/NVQ's, while social workers and occupational therapists have their professional qualifications. It is thought that the presumed difference in educational levels might then require different approaches in the way the training is delivered.

I suggest that a much more significant distinction lies in the different contexts within which the records are written. Each group records for different purposes. Direct care workers record on the basis of their regular observation and monitoring of service users' day-to-day health and well-being as part of the ongoing care they provide. It was for this group that the previous manual *For the Record* was largely written. In contrast social workers and occupational therapists, as care managers, record for the purpose of assessment. They are required to identify the service user's social care needs, write the care plan from those identified needs, and make a sufficiently effective case for the allocation of specific resources.

It's All in the Record is aimed primarily at those training care managers in case recording. The learning material in the manual is relevant for those working in adult services. The emphasis is on recording within the context of assessment. Social workers and care managers are involved in collecting information about a service user from various sources, and then producing a coherent account of that person's needs at a specific point in time. They are required to reflect the service user's views and accurately describe the person's situation, in order to ensure that the appropriate services are made available.

Although the main emphasis in this second manual is on case recording undertaken by care managers, a section is also included which will be relevant for those training domiciliary care workers in recording. This manual is concerned with trying to achieve a better understanding of how to support workers in open recording. Domiciliary workers are in the front-line in relation to this issue. Unlike any other group of workers, they are expected to record on their own, at the end of a very time-limited visit to a service user, and without the opportunity to reflect on what they might write. They are expected to write a meaningful communication to the next colleague who will be visiting that service user, while at the same time aware that what they write can be immediately read by the service user, the user's family and any other visitor to the house. This manual provides practical guidance in how they can be effectively supported in this demanding task.

Why do you need it?

The problem with case recording

Case recording for care managers is a central activity. Unlike direct care workers, the effectiveness of care managers is largely judged through the written record. The case record is the account of their work and so it becomes the main source of evidence for evaluating their performance. Joint reviews and inspections in many different authorities, as well as a succession of enquiries have highlighted case recording as a problem. Many of the criticisms suggest concerns over practice:

- Service led rather than needs led assessments.
- Assessments are not focused on outcomes.
- Assessments are not holistic and emphasise weaknesses and deficits.
- Lack of evidence for decisions taken.
- Insufficient analysis of information.
- The service user's voice is not heard.
- Fact and opinion are not always distinguished.

It is not clear however, whether these criticisms identify shortcomings in the way practitioners actually work, or whether the problems lie in the way practitioners describe their work in the case record. Nor is it clear whether the problems in recording practice arise from a lack of skill, or from trying to resolve a series of potentially competing demands in the case recording process. One of the major difficulties workers face is the need to write for a number of different audiences, e.g. service users, carers, managers, other professionals, resource allocation panels, direct care providers. All of these different readerships have their own expectations.

- How do you write in language the service user will understand, but still produce an assessment which will maintain your own professional credibility in the eyes of colleagues from other agencies and disciplines?
- How do you highlight a service user's strengths and still make an effective case for the required resources to support that individual?
- How do you record the sometimes conflicting views of service users and carers and still respect confidentiality?
- How do you provide an accurate account which may leave yourself or your department open to questions of liability?

Case recording is a complex and difficult business and yet it remains something of a 'Cinderella' in the repertoire of professional skills. The skills of case recording are rarely formally taught. Often practitioners, both long established and recently qualified, will say that the only guidance they received on recording was in their practice placements. So case recording is learned from practitioners who themselves did not receive any tuition, other than in their own placements.

Single (England), unified (Wales) or single shared (Scotland) assessment

An important impetus for training in recording and assessment skills has been the move towards single/shared or unified assessment. This represents the most significant development in adult service provision since the introduction of 'community care'. Social service departments and health authorities, as well as other public sector services, will be required to work more collaboratively. Assessments will be undertaken by a variety of practitioners from different disciplines and from different agencies. An 'overview assessment' will involve the care co-ordinator assessing and recording needs which may go beyond their normal area of expertise. Those assessments will then be shared with all those involved in working with that service user. Single or unified assessment will necessitate much closer and more co-operative working between agencies, and the recorded assessment will be central in this process.

It will be vital that practitioners are competent and confident in recording assessments that are effective across agency and professional boundaries.

Many of the principles of single/shared or unified assessment echo the criticisms that have been made of case recording. Practitioners are encouraged to ensure that:

- Service users' views are central to the assessment process.
- Assessments should provide a rounded picture of an individual's needs, as well as identifying strengths and abilities.
- Assessments should focus on outcomes.
- Assessments should provide clear evidence for the decisions reached.

Single/shared or unified assessment provides an opportunity to reflect on current practice in relation to recording and assessment. Its successful implementation will depend on many factors, but an important one will be practitioners, who understand and are able to meet the expectations being placed on them.

Related issues

Writing skills

Many people still expect recording training to address the issue of writing skills. Even for practitioners who have gone through professional training, there are still sometimes concerns over their ability to express themselves in writing. Issues of spelling, punctuation and grammar are identified as problem areas. While these issues often preoccupy managers, there is already an adequate supply of training material to meet these learning needs and so they are not specifically addressed in this manual. A clear and precise use of language is underlined in all the demonstrated examples of good recording practice throughout the manual, but a key message is that a record can be well written and perfectly punctuated and still be a poor record, because it fails to achieve its purpose.

This is because recording also includes the ability to structure and organise information. While difficulties in this area may arise from a lack of competence in using written English, the source of the problem is usually a failure to understand the basic purpose of the written record. Confusion around the purpose of the record then often results in muddled thinking and a failure to identify the main issues. Information is given, but there is no logic to how the points are related. What is the record trying to achieve and who is it for?

Answering these questions helps to establish the relevance of different information, and suggests how to present it in order to communicate your message most effectively. The manual does address these more fundamental questions. The last chapter specifically addresses the challenge of writing for a number of different readerships in the same record.

Legal issues

The manual explores in some detail the implications for practitioners of the Data Protection Act. This piece of legislation has caused much confusion in many agencies. Practitioners involved in case recording, who regularly share information with colleagues both within and outside of their own organisation, are often left vulnerable as to what is acceptable within the Act. The material is designed to explore those areas where the interpretation of the law is less clear.

The manual does not attempt to address the specific legal requirements of child protection or mental health work. These have their own particular legal frameworks which go beyond the scope of this manual.

The manual does, however, make it clear that all recording should be written as though it might be used as evidence in a court of law. Workers sometimes admit that they are more careful in their recording of certain cases, because they see them as potentially difficult and likely to be the subject of dispute. It is impossible, however, to predict what might happen in the life of a particular case. Even those cases that appear straightforward and unproblematic may take an unexpected turn, leaving the worker wondering how well their record will stand up to scrutiny, and how far it complies with the rules of evidence. The manual demonstrates how to ensure such standards are met in all recordings.

Anti-oppressive issues and recording

It would be impossible to focus on recording and not confront the way in which language can be used to reinforce negative assumptions and stereotypical attitudes. Language can be used oppressively. Its influence is subtle and its effect can be insidious. Through language we can describe reality in such a way that our view is taken to be the only view, or at least the only reasonable view. Service users are often at a disadvantage in their confidence and competence in using language, and so may find it difficult to challenge or put forward an alternative account of their situation to the one the practitioner has given.

These issues underpin the entire manual. Every case study and exercise is designed to help practitioners reflect on the power of language and how it can be misused to maintain a power imbalance between the service user and themselves. Practitioners are encouraged to look at how they can address that imbalance through more accurate and inclusive recording.

It is acknowledged that specific groups are often further disadvantaged in our society by virtue of their race, religion, gender, sexual orientation, age, social class, disability etc. While the manual does not attempt to explain systematically why and how specific groups may experience less power and influence in society than others, case studies are included to illustrate the particular issues which may arise in trying to accurately record the perspective of individuals belonging to such groups.

As in section on the cartoons and the caroonist, unless relevant, the ethnic origin of the people in the scenarios is not given. The UK has one of the highest rates of interracial marriage in the world, and nothing should be assumed about a person's ethnicity based solely on their name.

These issues are sometimes very complex. If we look at the example of Farah Ali Ahmed in Chapter 3, Farah came to Britain from Somalia as an asylum seeker. How much information do we need to know about Farah's background in Somalia and the circumstances of his flight from that country in order to understand his current situation?

He is the victim of an anti-Muslim attack and in the case history we learn that he has admitted to sometimes hitting his estranged wife. How do we interpret this information? We can look at it in terms of gender issues, which would emphasise his role as an oppressive male or we can look at it in terms of his cultural background, which may or may not involve particular beliefs and attitudes about the rights of married men in relation to their wives. We could also look at it in terms of someone who has been tortured and endured so many extreme adversities that his behaviour is seen as evidence of despair and the breakdown of his own coping mechanisms.

The manual will underline the importance of recording the service user's story in their own terms, describing their understanding of their experience. We need to hear their account in the record, and only when we have ensured that their voice is heard should we go on to include our own professional interpretation. It is inevitable that when we are trying to record the stories of service users, who belong to groups or are in circumstances far removed from our own experience and what we would regard as familiar, we are faced with a greater challenge.

Preconceptions and our tendency to see the person in terms of their membership of a particular disadvantaged group may make it difficult to hear their individual story. Instead their story is heard through the filter of our assumptions and expectations in relation to that group. Unwittingly we may focus on those parts of the story which reinforce our knowledge and understanding of such groups, and overlook the parts of the story that do not fit into that perspective.

Equally, we run the risk that, by ignoring the structural ways in which people have been disadvantaged in society, we leave out an important dimension to understanding their lives and circumstances. If we simply listen to the individual stories of people who have a physical disability, without also being aware of the way in which society, rather than their disability, has effectively marginalised them, then we simply add to that very partial view and so further reinforce the marginal position of this group of people.

The manual also addresses the often overlooked area of how service users may be discriminated against simply as a consequence of the practitioner's implicit disapproval or dislike of them, their values, habits, beliefs or practices.

In Chapter 1 we meet Mr Martin Heiberg, who is a wheelchair user, following a hunt-riding accident. During the transcript of the interview between the care manager and Mr Heiberg, we discover that Mr Heiberg has behaved abusively towards the home care workers who have been visiting him. Many people might find Mr Heiberg's manner rude and unpleasant. They might also have feelings about the circumstances of his accident, dependent on their views about blood sports. However, the message of the exercise is that, despite any feelings of disapproval that might be roused by Mr Heiberg, the most important objective of the recording is to provide an accurate account of what has been said during the interview. The account should be one that Mr Heiberg would recognise. It should also provide the reader with sufficient information to understand the views and positions stated by both Mr Heiberg and the care manager.

While stressing the importance of hearing the service user's story, it has to be acknowledged that where English is either a second language for a service user, or they are solely dependent on an interpreter, it may be more difficult to always ensure that the service user and worker have understood one another sufficiently for an accurate record to be possible. When the communication between user and worker is conducted through an interpreter, this intermediary may introduce their own subtle nuances of meaning in the way they are understanding and then conveying what is being said by each party. This may happen irrespective of the interpreter's competence with each of the languages being spoken.

Similarly, where service users, because of some communication problem such as aphasia, are dependent on relatives to speak for them, it should always be acknowledged that this is the carer's interpretation of what they think the service user is saying. Whilst care should be taken to ensure the service user's views are being accurately expressed, it is sometimes very easy for a carer to become so much the voice of the service user, that the service user may find it difficult to assume their own separate and distinct voice.

These different issues point to the essence of the manual. When we record we are trying to describe and reflect someone else's reality. We are hampered by our own selective perception and our tendency to construct reality in terms we understand and with which we are familiar. Even with an awareness and a concern to act in a way which does not oppress or discriminate, it is still sometimes difficult to recognise the extent to which our own way of making sense of the world may, without our realising, ignore or invalidate someone else's way, simply because it is so removed from the world to which we are accustomed and regard as normal.

The principle of anti-oppressive practice is to respect all service users, whatever their culture, background or experience. A great deal has been written about the discrimination of groups on the basis of gender, ethnicity and disability for example, but these are only examples and it follows that there is no definitive or exclusive checklist of categories which require special attention to mitigate the risk of anti-oppressive practice.

Agency forms and systems

The manual is concerned with general principles of good recording practice, and does not attempt to address the particular paper forms or computerised systems employed by different departments. While practitioners clearly need to understand how to use such systems, there is a danger that recording is seen as little more than form-filling. Assessment then becomes an administrative chore rather than an exercise of professional skill. The manual is concerned to emphasise the professional nature of the recording and assessment process.

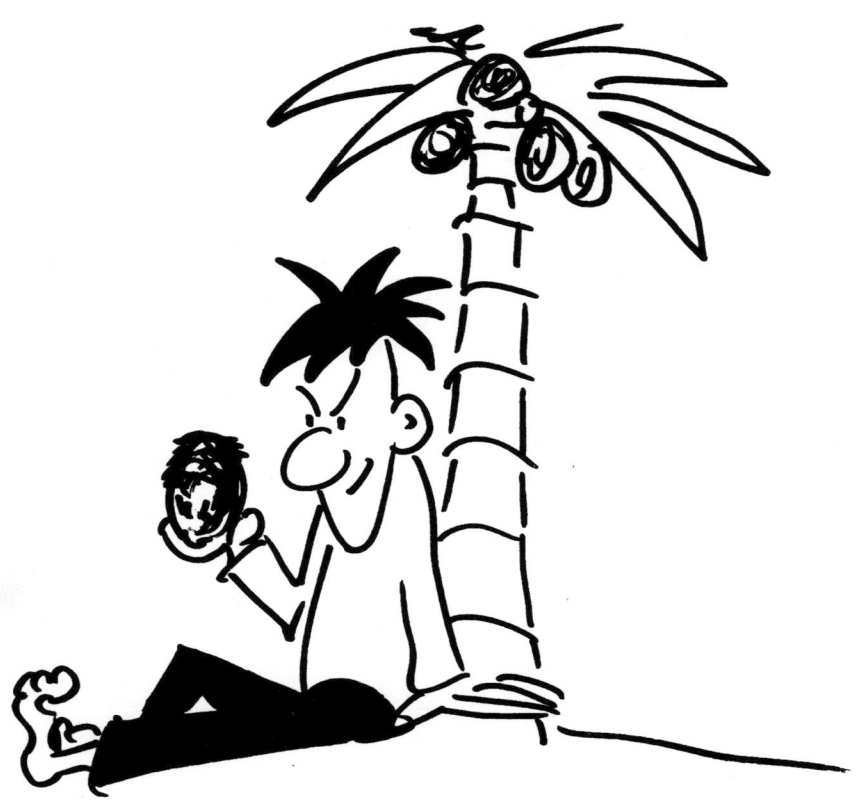

In a nutshell

It's all in the Record explores the challenge of open recording and addresses the criticisms that have been made of case recording practice. It is designed to increase practitioner confidence in a task that many find frustrating and confusing.

The manual is divided into five chapters. Each chapter focuses on a particular set of issues in recording. The chapters then go on to provide exercises which are designed to help practitioners explore these issues and further develop their recording practice.

Chapter 1: Telling it Like it is

The first chapter addresses the central issue of how we accurately describe reality, when our perception of any situation is necessarily selective. How do we use language, which conveys such subtlety of meaning, to construct a coherent account and to ensure that our account will be understood in the way we intended? It is important to establish a basic understanding of this fundamental issue in recording. Exercises have been devised to stimulate awareness of the difficulty we all have in providing accurate and factual accounts of what we have observed and heard.

What did you say?

Transcript exercises have been devised to encourage workers to explore how they make judgements about what is relevant to record from a discussion with a service user, and how accurately their record reflects what the service user actually said. They are designed to raise particular questions about how far our feelings toward the service user may influence our perceptions, and the subsequent account of the discussion we have had with them.

'A medical opinion is a fact'

The above statement was made, in all seriousness, by a participant on a recording skills course. It provides an insight into the confusion that still exists between what constitutes fact and what constitutes opinion. The issue goes way beyond the simple requirement to use the preface, 'In my opinion'. The section looks at how opinions can often masquerade as facts. It explores the way in which language can be used to present assumptions, speculation, distortions and exaggerations as factual statements of self-evident truth.

Chapter 2: We Know Just What You Need

This chapter focuses on the assessment process and the way in which that process is recorded. As indicated earlier there are considerable questions as to where and how the problems in assessments arise, but the exercises are designed to encourage learners to reflect on the process as a whole.

The recording of assessments for many workers has become an administrative chore, where forms are filled and boxes ticked with a sense of dull resignation. It has become a paper exercise rather than a meaningful way of understanding and meeting someone's needs. Care managers routinely complain that they cannot include all the information they feel they should, because 'the box isn't big enough'. This seems a classic example of the tools being allowed to drive the process. So the point of the exercise becomes the completion of the form, rather than an accurate assessment of someone's needs. The chapter attempts to get beyond the narrow concerns of how to complete particular forms, and instead encourages practitioners to look at the wider picture; what is the purpose of an assessment, what is it trying to achieve and how do we ensure our recording assists that purpose?

Whose need is it anyway?

This section is designed to explore how easily practitioners adopt a service led approach to assessments without even realising it. The exercise involves an extended case study, where practitioners are required to conduct an assessment interview and to identify the service user's needs from that interview.

We know where we're going

One of the greatest sources of difficulty and frustration described by practitioners is how to write outcome objectives from identified needs. There is a feeling that this involves nothing more than unnecessary repetition. Practitioners seem to genuinely flounder because they have not been given any useful guidance on how to distinguish needs from objectives. When this material has been included in training sessions practitioners are clearly relieved that finally there is some practical explanation on how to write objectives, which then provides them with a greater understanding and insight into what is involved in writing a care plan.

Chapter 3: The Bus Principle

This chapter refers to the proverbial bus, under which practitioners are reminded they may one day fall, and asked how adequate their records would be, in that event, for anyone else to pick up and work with.

It's a long story

This is concerned with the problem of intuitive recording, where the practitioner only tells part of the story in the case record. Because they know it so well they have difficulty in viewing it from the perspective of the reader, who does not have all the background information in their head. The material is designed to encourage learners to think about how much information is necessary to tell the story effectively for the purpose of the record.

It's obvious isn't it?

This again focuses on the problem of the case record only providing a partial account. It looks particularly at why practitioners do not always sufficiently analyse the information they provide, and why they often neglect to provide a clear explanation or adequate evidence for the decisions made.

Intuitive recording is often part of the problem, but practitioners have also become less confident about providing any analysis in the case record. They feel, often mistakenly, that by sticking to a purely descriptive record, they are keeping to the facts, on which they are less likely to be challenged. This then extends to not always explaining why or how decisions have been made. A classic example of this is the entry in the case file reading, 'No further action required', as though the record, along with agency intervention needs no more input. But the question is left hanging: why was it decided that no further action was needed? The material will stimulate learners to reflect on the issues and questions not addressed in a descriptive record.

Chapter 4: I'd Like to Tell You But . . .

This chapter is specifically concerned with the issue of open recording and how comfortable we are to share information with service users. It inevitably includes references to the Data Protection Act. However, it tries to go beyond a simple legalistic interpretation of the Act. It sets in context the legal provisions by explaining how the Act should be practically applied in the workplace. It explores how we collect and use information about service users, and examines the implications for both practice and recording.

Open and above board

The way in which we record often reflects our approach to practice. What and how we write about service users reveals a lot about the way we work with them. Do we view them as detached objects of interest to be observed and commented upon, or do we view them as partners in a collaborative process? Most practitioners would subscribe to the latter, and yet their recording does not always suggest an inclusive approach. The material will encourage learners to recognise how the record reflects practice and suggest how to ensure a more inclusive way of working.

We know better

This section focuses on the use of the 'restricted information category' in the case file, looking at when and in what circumstances it might be appropriate. It deals particularly with how we record information which relates to knowledge, insights, or understandings we might have about the service user, but which we may feel the service user is not yet ready to hear. How, for example, do we record a situation where the service user is dependent on a carer, the carer is diagnosed with a terminal illness, and neither are able or willing to talk about the implications for them both? These are difficult dilemmas, both for practice and for how we record. The material is designed to help learners explore how they might record in these problematic circumstances.

For all to see

This section specifically addresses the needs of domiciliary care workers, and examines the difficult task of maintaining a record in the service user's own home. This raises issues about what and how you record, given that what is written can be immediately read by the service user, their family and potentially, anyone visiting the house. The record has implications for the ongoing relationship between the worker and service user, as well as the protection and security of the service user. The material is designed to help domiciliary care workers to record effectively in this demanding situation.

Have you heard?

This looks at how we share information with other professionals, particularly those working in other agencies, exploring particularly the issues around the use of third party information. It also raises the question of how we work in an inclusive way with service users, protect their confidentiality, and still share necessary information with other agencies. These issues will become more pressing with the move towards single assessment.

The material is designed to help learners think about how they share information with other agencies, and how they use information given to them by third parties.

Chapter 5: You Can't Please All of the People All of the Time

As mentioned earlier, one of the fundamental problems for care managers and social workers is how to record for a variety of readerships. The chapter examines how practitioners' perceptions of the expectations of different audiences influence the way in which they write the record. It brings together some of the issues from the earlier chapters and helps to explore the dilemmas that practitioners routinely face in their recording and suggests strategies for resolving them.

Guidance in using the manual

To help you navigate around the manual the various activities or materials have been assigned their own particular icon. At the start of each training exercise you will find:

↗ The objective of the exercise.

🕐 The time required for the exercise.

✎ The materials required to run the exercise.

ⓘ Trainer's guidelines in running the exercise.

At the end of the exercises are the special materials that you will need to run that particular exercise:

oht Overhead transparencies (OHTs)

▤ Handouts (HOs)

✓ Exercise sheets

While the exercises do contain 'trainer's guidelines' in respect of timing, these are approximate and can vary depending on the size of the group and the degree to which they engage in discussion. We have tried to produce material which can be used by experienced trainers and by those, including many managers, who are not so experienced in the training role. The guidelines are there to provide a basis for planning and organising a programme, but the manual can be used in as flexible a way as needed. Some exercises could be used in a one-to-one supervision session and some can be used within the context of a team meeting.

We have included fairly detailed notes of the points we believe should be included in feedback and discussion as well as providing 'model' or 'suggested' records for certain exercises. These are not necessarily meant to be definitive, but they offer anyone using the manual some indication of what the record should look like. Such 'suggested' recordings should be regarded as a guide rather than the 'correct' or 'prescribed' answer.

Chapter 1: Telling it Like it is

Section A: Introduction

This is the fundamental dilemma in recording. How do we accurately describe our experience, when that experience is shared by other people, who will have their own perception of what happened, and their own way of describing their experience? This is covered to some degree in *For the Record* in Section 3 on *Selective Perception*.

It is curious how many people, who have gone through professional training or been exposed to the ideas of social science, will understand the idea of relative realities in a theoretical sense, and yet will act in the everyday world as though there is an absolute version of reality, which is invariably their own.

The very exposure to professional knowledge will lead us to believe that we do indeed have a more informed insight and understanding, which we are expected to use in describing our observations and experience. So, on the one hand, there is the awareness that we live in a relative world, and yet on the other, we are still expected to function as experts in terms of our own sphere of knowledge.

It is not surprising that these tensions are often put to one side in the practical business of getting on with the job. Everyone is under more and more pressure, and the emphasis is on results, getting the job done. So it is hardly surprising that workers can easily lapse into seeing their accounts of other people as unproblematic. Recording is regarded as an administrative chore, a necessary evil. The awkward question of how we reconcile different versions of reality into one coherent account is not often addressed.

This is not the place to enter into a philosophical debate about these issues, interesting as that may be to pursue. The purpose of this manual is to offer practical guidance. Learners will be provided with experiences which will

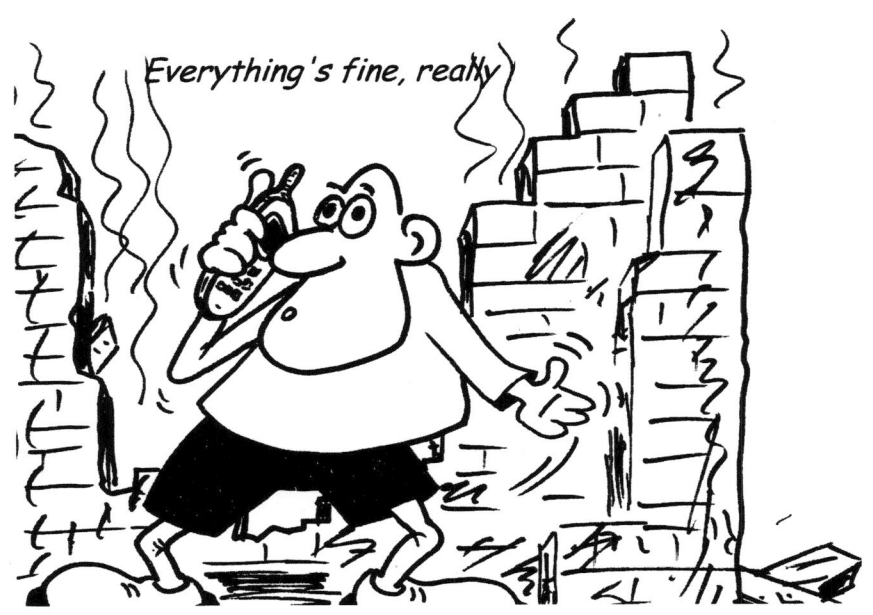

encourage them to reflect on the taken for granted way in which we normally make sense of our experience, and how all of us are constantly trying to engage and negotiate with each other's constructions of reality.

Before we go on to the specific sections, there are two introductory exercises. The first explores the theme of how either one individual may be seen quite differently by the various people who know them, or how one individual can give different accounts of their feelings and attitudes to different people. This is developed further in the second exercise where a description of an individual is gradually revealed, and learners are asked to reflect on their reactions to the different pieces of information given, and how their feelings toward the person are affected as the picture unfolds.

✔️ Exercise 1: Telling stories

↗️ Objective

To explore the ways in which people construct different accounts of themselves and other people and how those accounts can be reconciled into a coherent understanding.

🕐 Time

Allow 40 minutes for this exercise

✏️ Materials

- Flipchart paper
- Marker pens for each group
- Blu tack or masking tape
- HO 1a, 1b, 1c and 1d: Isabel Seymour, or HO 2a, 2b and 2c: Clive Meeks

ⓘ Trainer's guidelines

Step 1: allow 5 minutes
Introduce the exercise. Split the group into smaller groups. With 'Isabel Seymour' ensure that there are at least four members to each group. With 'Clive Meeks' ensure that there are at least three members to each group. Give each group a piece of flipchart paper and a pen.

With 'Isabel Seymour' give each of the 'stories', HO 1a: 'Alec's story', HO 1b: 'Miriam's story', HO 1c: 'Amy's story' and HO 1d: 'Nora's story' to a different member of each group. In groups of five or six, two people will need to read the same story. The exercise depends on different group members only reading one of the stories. They are then asked to write on the flipchart paper one description

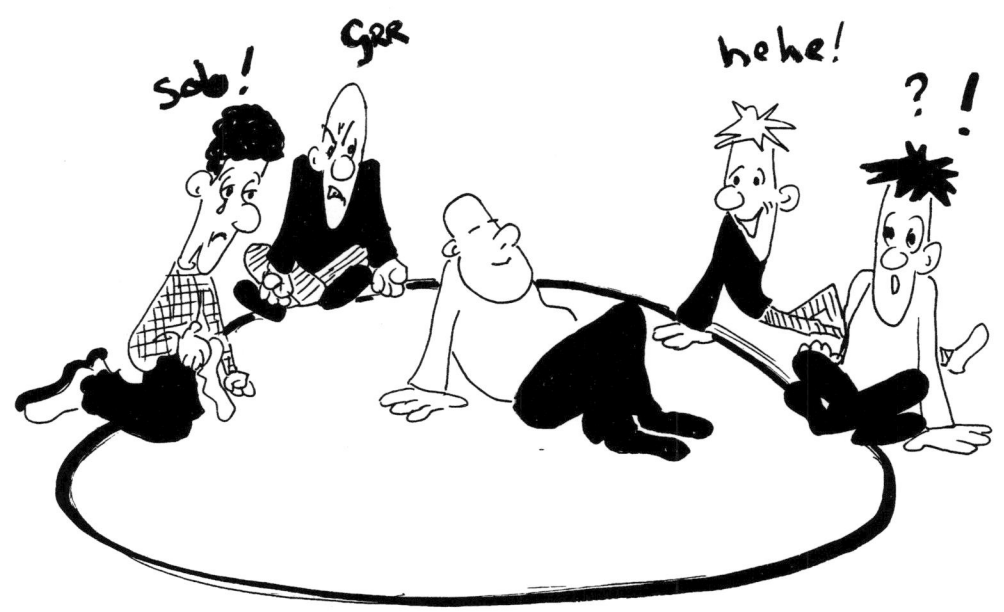

of Isabel. They are asked to share information from their different accounts, but not to show other group members their particular story.

With 'Clive Meeks', give each of the accounts given by Clive, HO 2a: his home carer Rita, HO 2b: daughter Megan and HO 2c: son Derek, to a different member of each group. Again it may be necessary, depending on numbers, for two people to share the same account. In the same way as 'Isabel Seymour', the exercise depends on different group members only reading one of the accounts. Ask participants to write on flipchart paper one account of Clive's attitudes and feelings, but not to show other group members their particular story.

Step 2: allow 20 minutes
Groups work on producing one account.

Step 3: allow 15 minutes
Put the completed pieces of flipchart paper on the wall and ask each group to describe the process they went through in producing their description. Ask them whether they felt it was possible to come up with one definitive description of Isabel through the accounts given by other people, or one definitive account of Clive's attitude and feelings.

HO 1a: Isabel Seymour: Alec's story (Isabel's ex-husband)

Isabel and I met at a friend's party. I really thought she was out of my league. She was incredibly attractive and very confident. She'd just graduated and was talking of becoming an actress. I was in my first year of teaching. I know I'd just drifted into teaching because I couldn't think of anything else to do. Well I had fancied myself as a journalist, but I never thought I'd get into that. I mean I didn't want to have to work on local rags, covering the latest WI fund-raising event. If I was going to be a journalist, then I wanted to work on a serious paper, or better still, television. But I didn't have the connections, and if I'm honest, I didn't have the confidence. I've never had what you call people skills. I'm just not very diplomatic. I can't pretend.

But Isabel seemed to get on with people so easily. Where I'd be awkward and wary, she'd be straight in there, really warm and genuine. I suppose it was a case of opposites attract. She got a lot of stick from her friends and family, because no one could see what she saw in me. But it didn't seem to matter. She said we were meant for each other – soul-mates.

But things changed after Paul and Amy came along. She just became totally pre-occupied with them. I know Paul was difficult, but whenever I tried to help, she told me I made things worse. We just seemed to drift further and further apart. My job was becoming more demanding, bringing work home and all that, but she never minded, because she never seemed to notice whether I was there or not.

I loved the kids but I sometimes felt I was intruding, like she'd created this ideal little world for her and Paul and Amy, and she didn't want anyone to disturb it. She never really liked them going to school. We never really rowed much. We just became indifferent to one another.

When I met Julie, it was like someone was breathing life back into me. I suppose I thought, first of all, that I could see Julie and still stay with Isabel and the kids. But Julie said she couldn't settle for that and faced me with an ultimatum. I'd got to the point where I couldn't give her up and life with Isabel was just so empty.

I felt terrible about the kids, but I thought Isabel and I could work something out, so I could still see them regularly. But she just seemed to go off her head. She made it so difficult for me to see them that in the end, I thought I was causing them more grief by trying to stay in contact. And when Julie got this job in Australia, I decided to go with her. I know Isabel's got herself in a bit of a mess, because I still hear about her through the friend, at whose party we first met.

I feel bad, but I've made a new life for myself out here. Julia's pregnant and I think my first responsibility now is to her and the baby.

HO 1b: Isabel Seymour: Miriam's story (Isabel's friend)

I've known Isabel ever since we were at university together. That's nearly twenty years ago now. She always seemed so confident. She had strong opinions on everything, and wasn't afraid to express them. But she is a very kind person really. She was always ready to listen to other people's problems. She can be very emotional, she's quite sensitive if someone criticises her.

We met through the drama society. She was studying psychology and I was studying history. She was a very good actress, a lot better than me. She usually got the lead parts. She could have turned professional. I think she did consider it, but then she got mixed up with that Alec. I never liked him, he always seemed so dominating. Isabel became quieter, more subdued after she met him. She said he was different when he was with her. She had always seemed so independent, and yet after he came along, she seemed to slip into the role of the dutiful wife.

She worked part-time at that day centre for people with psychiatric problems, but the kids always came first. She doted on those two children, and the older one, Paul, was a real handful. She had a lot of problems with him, when he was younger. I didn't think Alec was much help, although he always made out he knew everything.

I wasn't surprised when he ran off with that other woman. They were teachers in the same school. Isabel put a brave face on it. I kept telling her I thought she was better off without him. I know it wasn't a good age as far as the children were concerned, both of them in their teens. They became very resentful. There wasn't very much money and teenagers can be very cruel.

Isabel threw herself into all that political stuff. I think it was all a bit too much. She was working full-time by then with a project for refugees. I think she was trying to sort everyone else's problems even if she couldn't sort out her own.

I saw the breakdown coming. She was just living on her nerves. I know she's supposed to be getting better now, but she's not the woman she was. She's been talking about moving to Ireland, where her father's family originally came from. But she doesn't know anyone there. The children don't want to go. They said they'll carry on living with their Gran. She's been looking after them since their Mum went into hospital.

But Isabel just seems to be shutting everyone out now. We used to see each other quite regularly, but ever since her breakdown, it's really difficult to get to see her. It's like she can't be bothered with anyone anymore.

HO 1c: Isabel Seymour: Amy's story (Isabel's daughter)

Mum and I get on O.K., I guess. It's been more difficult since her breakdown. She was acting so weird before she went into hospital. My brother and I were really worried, but we didn't know what to do. Gran was great. She got the doctor, and he persuaded Mum that she really needed someone to look after her. We've been living with Gran since then, and now Mum's talking about moving to Ireland, Paul and I have decided to stay with Gran. We just don't know where we are with Mum anymore.

After the divorce she was never home, she was either working or out fund-raising or canvassing or something. It was a really bad time. Paul and I wanted to see our Dad, but Mum got really upset whenever we mentioned him.

When we were young, she'd always been there for us. She was brilliant. She was really funny and made everything special. She'd make up games for us to play. She'd know how you were feeling even without you saying anything. Friends used to say they wished they had a Mum more like ours. Paul used to be very naughty, but Mum would always know how to calm him down.

It's funny I don't really remember any rows between Mum and Dad. Just one day he was gone and we didn't know why. Well Mum said he'd gone off with this other woman, and when we saw him, he said how he still loved us and nothing would ever change that, but we still don't really understand why he and Mum split up. I mean they didn't seem that bad together.

Anyway it all feels a bit of a mess now. We haven't heard anything from Dad since he moved abroad and neither of us can talk to Mum anymore. We're just really glad we've got Gran.

HO 1d: Isabel Seymour: Nora's story (Isabel's mother)

Isabel was always highly strung as a child. She was very jealous of her brother. He was born just after she started school. I thought she would be old enough to enjoy helping to look after a baby brother, but I could never trust her with him. There could be quite a spiteful side to her, when she felt she wasn't the centre of attention.

But she was always very bright. Her father always thought she would go far. He used to spoil her. Fathers always do. So I had to be the disciplinarian and Isabel didn't always like that. She could be very headstrong sometimes.

We were both very proud when she got to university, although we didn't see much of her after she got there. Her father was quite hurt by that but he wouldn't say anything. He missed her a lot, but she was always too busy with this and that, to visit us very often.

Of course we had our doubts about that Alec. He thought a lot of himself, but she wouldn't hear a word against him. She was determined to marry him, no matter what we said. But after the kids came along, she just became besotted with them. Her world just revolved around them. That's why she had so many problems with Paul. I never did like Alec, but he didn't get a look in after those children arrived. Men will only put up with so much, and if temptation is put their way, well it's happened plenty of times before.

But Isabel would never forgive him. I said to her that I thought it was important for Paul and Amy's sake that she and Alec sorted things out so that even if they split up the kids wouldn't end up feeling pulled between them. But it all got very messy and Isabel did make it very difficult for the children to see their father. I didn't think that was right and I told her so.

Then she took on all that work. She said she had to because Alec didn't give her enough money. But she drove herself into the ground with all that extra work with the Labour Party. She didn't have to do all that. So I wasn't surprised when she had the breakdown. Of course I had Paul and Amy. I know I'm on my own now and getting on a bit, but I told her I'd look after the children until she got better.

But now she's got this mad idea about going off to Ireland. The kids don't want to go and I think she should consider them. I've told her I think she's being selfish, but she's never listened to me. She'll end up going on her own and I don't think that's going to do anybody any good.

HO 2a: Clive Meeks

Clive Meeks is a 79-year-old white man, who has lived on his own since his wife, Lilly, died two years ago. He has had a series of small strokes in the last year which have left him more frail. He has a home carer visit twice a day to help him get up and go to bed. He has two children, Megan aged 52, who lives alone and runs a small charity concerned with the homeless, and Derek, aged 47 who works as a finance clerk with the council and is married to Jill and they have three children.

Clive has been visited recently by his friend Harold, aged 81.

Imagine the following information being given by Clive to his:

Home carer: Rita

It made a change seeing my friend Harold yesterday. He only visits when his son brings him to Manchester. John was here for some conference and drove his Dad down so he could come and see me. He always was a nice boy John, very considerate. I told Harold he was lucky to still have his wife and to have kids that put themselves out for him. That was always the way. Harold was the lucky one. I've known him since we were in the army together. They used to say you'd be alright if you were with Harold, 'cause he's lucky. Me, I've never been lucky. I mean I haven't had a bad life, but it's been a slog all the way. I haven't got anything that I haven't had to work hard for.

Lilly was my biggest stroke of luck. I did alright there. My Mum said that I should grab her before someone else snapped her up. At the time I wasn't sure whether I was ready to settle down. But she got pregnant and, well, in them days you didn't have much choice, you had to get married. Life's funny like that. The best thing that has happened in my life was an accident. I suppose to begin with, when Megan was still a baby, I still had my doubts, but she was a sweet kid and always into mischief, but they change you know. When she got to be a teenager we had nothing but trouble, always arguing about this and that. I thought she'd settle down eventually, but she was too independent that one. It's not done her any good. She's never been able to keep a man. And now what's she got, nothing.

Derek on the other hand was always a quiet one. But he married that Jill. They say opposites attract. She was quite a 'looker', and she could turn on the charm when she wanted to. She takes people in, but she's really only out for herself. Lilly always said that if anything happened to her, she knew I'd be alright, because Derek and Jill would look after me. Jill was supposed to have said to her once that she didn't need to worry about me. Well that was a bloody lie.

☐ HO 2b: Clive Meeks

Clive Meeks is 79 and has lived on his own since his wife, Lilly died two years ago. He has had a series of small strokes in the last year which have left him more frail. He has a home carer visit twice a day to help him get up and go to bed. He has two children, Megan aged 52, who lives alone and runs a small charity concerned with the homeless, and Derek, aged 47 who works as a finance clerk with the council and is married to Jill and they have three children.

Clive has been visited recently by his friend Harold, aged 81.

Imagine the following information being given by Clive to his:

Daughter: Megan

I keep telling you, you'll wear yourself out with that job, but you never listen. I've had Harold to visit in the last week. He's looking well. He said June's taken up painting. A bloody daft thing to do at her age, but Harold reckons it's good for her, gives her an interest. He said that's what I needed, an interest. He always was a bit keen to give people the benefit of his advice. I told him I was doing alright as I was and I didn't need any 'interest'.

Derek was over last Sunday. He said he's not been well. He said he'd been getting these pains in his chest. I told him he should see the doctor, but he's too scared. Typical. You'd think that wife of his would tell him, but reading between the lines, I don't think things are too good there. I'm not surprised, she's never at home from what I can gather. The kids are left to fend for themselves. Derek said he doesn't see them, they're always off somewhere. I'd never be surprised to see her going off with someone else. He did look bad. I told him he shouldn't be going in to work if he was feeling that ill, but he said he was worried about people being made redundant, and he didn't want to give them any excuses to get rid of him.

They've changed the home help again. I've got another new one, Rita she's called. She's alright, but they come and go so quickly you don't know where you are with them. She's a bit young this one, looks like she's just come out of school. It's a funny job for a youngster, but at least she's a bit more lively than the last one.

I don't mind if you want to come for Christmas. It will make a nice change. I didn't enjoy last year at Derek and Jill's. She had her family over and I can't stand them.

HO 2c: Clive Meeks

Clive Meeks is 79 and has lived on his own since his wife, Lilly died two years ago. He has had a series of small strokes in the last year which have left him more frail. He has a home carer visit twice a day to help him get up and go to bed. He has two children, Megan aged 52, who lives alone and runs a small charity concerned with the homeless, and Derek, aged 47 who works as a finance clerk with the council and is married to Jill and they have three children.

Clive has been visited recently by his friend Harold, aged 81.

Imagine the following information being given by Clive to his:

Son: Derek

I'm glad to hear you're feeling a bit better. You had me worried when you were here last. They won't thank you at that bloody council. They'll get rid of you when it suits them. But you won't take any notice of me.

I saw my friend Harold recently. He came down for a visit. His son brought him, he was always a good lad. Harold's looking well, all things considered. I said it would be nice to be able to return the visit, but I couldn't see how I would be able to make it. I haven't seen his wife June for years. But I guess I'll just have to wait for John to bring his father down again sometime.

I spoke to Megan the other day. She says she wants to come and stay for Christmas. I don't know what's got into her. She doesn't usually do Christmas does she? Well, except to go and do good works for the undeserving poor. I suppose she's got wind that you and Jill are going to stay at some fancy hotel this year, and she's feeling guilty that her poor old Dad will be on his own. Well I suppose I ought to be suitably grateful. It's about time that she pulled her weight. She's left it to you for too long. Although I'm not standing for her vegetarian nonsense. I want a proper Christmas dinner. I'm sure she thinks she's going to have another go at me about moving into a home, but I've said to you, and I'll say it to her, 'I'd rather be dead'.

Exercise 2: Building up the picture

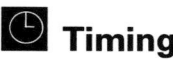 **Objective**

To explore how we can generalise and make assumptions from sometimes very limited information about people.

Timing

Allow 30 minutes for this exercise

Materials

- Case sheet: Anthony Singham
- or Case sheet: Sumitei Walker
- Pens and paper

Trainer's guidelines

Step 1: allow 1 minute
Introduce the exercise and ask participants to work in pairs. Explain that you will read out a series of statements about an individual. As each statement is read out, participants are asked to briefly discuss with their partner, their reaction to this new piece of information, and note on paper the main points they have discussed.

Step 2: allow 20 minutes
Read out each of the statements in turn, allowing approximately 30 seconds for the discussion and notes after the first statement, increasing the time by 10

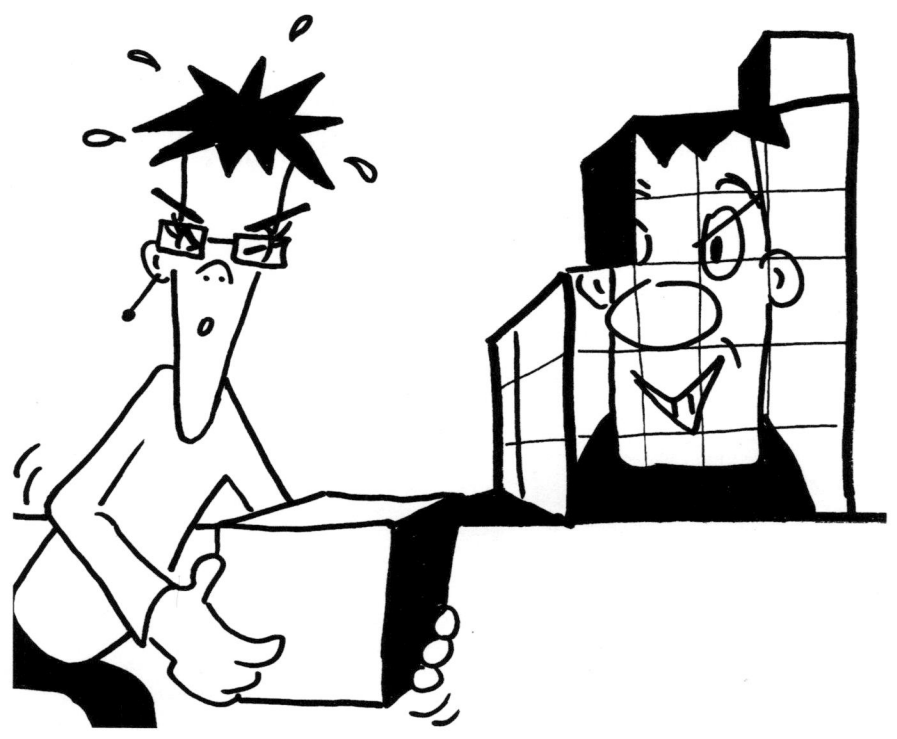

seconds after each succeeding statement. Allow at least 2 minutes for the discussion and final summarising after the last statement.

Step 3: allow 9 minutes

Ask each pair to summarise how their reactions developed to the succeeding information about the character. Draw out points about how we tend to make assumptions from limited information, and how we can find it difficult to reconcile seemingly contradictory information which does not fit with those assumptions.

Case sheet: Anthony Singham

1. Anthony was born in Malaysia 37 years ago.
2. He grew up in a Catholic orphanage after his mother abandoned him when he was 2 days old.
3. He came to England to study computing.
4. He gave up his studies and decided to become a priest.
5. He left the seminary after he developed schizophrenia.
6. He spent 5 years in and out of hospitals, sometimes living on the street.
7. When he was aged 31 he met a fellow patient during his stay in hospital. She was suffering from bi-polar disorder. They decided to get married.
8. He has not had any further hospital admissions and has helped care for his wife through 3 recurrences of her illness.
9. He now works as a web-site designer.
10. He is about to have a book of poetry published.

Case sheet: Sumitei Walker

1. Sumitei was born in Swindon 34 years ago, the eldest daughter of a Hindu family.
2. Her parents ran a dry cleaning business.
3. As a little girl she dreamed of being a ballet dancer when she grew up. She went to ballet classes until she was 16.
4. Her best friend at school died, aged 17, after taking Ecstasy.
5. She married a nurse.
6. Her brother is in jail for fraud.
7. She had a daughter 7 months ago.
8. She is on maternity leave and is being treated for post-natal depression.
9. She works as a GP.
10. Last week she stabbed her baby to death and then used the same knife to kill herself.

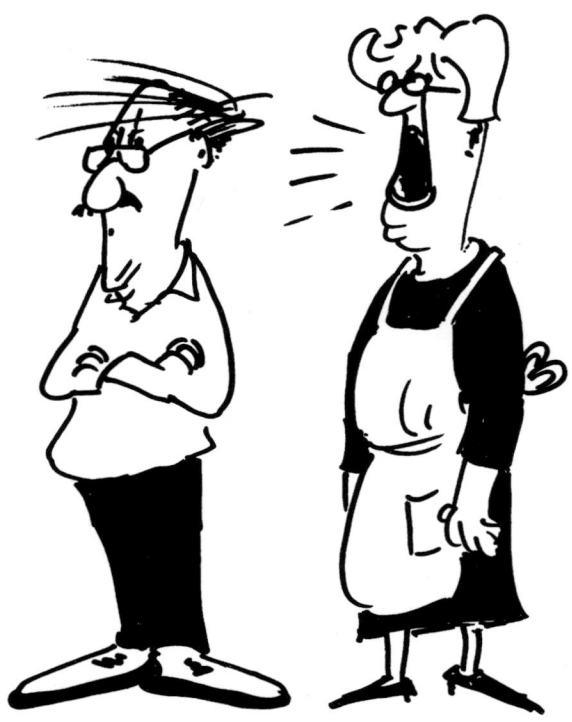

Section B: What did you say?

This section addresses the issue of how we summarise in the record the relevant information which has come from a discussion with a service user. The device of the transcript is being used. It is acknowledged that a transcript cannot include the information that would be conveyed through body language. However, it does provide a written record of exactly what was said, and it is interesting how, even with such a record, it is possible for the service user to be misquoted, or for the meaning of what was said to change in the way that a summary is then written.

Indeed, working with participants has provided a fascinating insight into how practitioners will spend considerable time in trying to construct a different form of words, in order to make a point that the service user has very clearly and adequately articulated in their own words.

The main message from this section is to let the service user's voice be heard; where appropriate quote, and always be careful, in any summary, that you do not distort or lose the meaning intended by the service user.

There are several transcripts to cover different service user groups. They are also designed to address the issue of how far our feelings toward the service user may influence the way we record. Martin Heiberg is deliberately written to provide an example of an, initially, very unsympathetic character, who some will regard as offensive. Much of what Fay Goldstein says may be seen as evidence of her confusion, so what sort of judgement is made about what is important or relevant to record, and what may we choose to disregard? Vincent Morris raises a number of issues. His situation is likely to evoke sympathy, as well as some frustration as to how much effective support we might be able to provide. There will be concern over the risk Vincent poses to himself. In addition there are difficulties about how much information can be shared with his partner. This last point will be addressed more fully in Chapter 4 when Vincent is the subject of a further exercise.

Exercise 3: Hearing the service user's voice

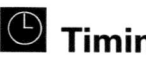 **Objective**

To encourage participants to record an accurate account of what has been discussed between a service user and a practitioner, enabling the service user's voice to be heard.

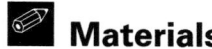 **Timing**

Allow 1 hour for this exercise

Materials

- Flipchart paper and marker pens
- Blu tack or masking tape
- HO 3: Martin Heiberg, or HO 4: Fay Goldstein, or HO 5: Vincent Morris

Optional – copies of suggested records, HO 3a, HO 4a or HO 5a

Trainer's guidelines

Step 1: allow 5 minutes
Introduce the exercise and divide the participants into groups of between two and four individuals. Give out the flipchart paper, pens and case-sheets of transcripts. Explain that the purpose of the exercise is not to evaluate or criticise the intervention of the practitioner. It is rather to provide an accurate and relevant record of what was said on the sheet of flipchart paper provided. Emphasise that they are expected to produce the actual record, not a set of headings or brief notes, simply indicating the points which should be included.

Step 2: allow 40 minutes
Participants to work together in writing the record from the transcript.

Step 3: allow 15 minutes
The completed sheets of flipchart paper should be put up on the wall and each group's record read out. The records can be compared in terms of what was included and how it was written. How far do the different records reflect what the service user said? It will be evident that different groups may adopt different formats and decide to structure the information in different ways. Some may follow a narrative style, others may organise the information under different headings. The point needs to be made that different formats can all be equally effective. The issue is not the format. It is the quality of the recorded information included in that format.

The suggested record can be provided as a HO or read out, but it may be more useful simply used as a guide for the trainer to draw out comparisons. What points were included and how were they recorded? Has there been any distortion of meaning? Are there any significant gaps?

HO 3: Transcript: Martin Heiberg, white

Martin, aged 55, and Martha Heiberg, aged 49, have been married for 25 years. Martin was involved in a hunt-riding accident three years ago. He has no movement below the waist. They have recently moved into the area for Martha to be nearer to her family. She originally met Martin while working in Germany.

A home care package was set up shortly after Martin moved into the area, involving two carers, calling twice a day. Martin is a large man, weighing 17 stone. Martha was diagnosed with angina five years ago. In the last three months, eight workers have said they are no longer prepared to visit Mr Heiberg. You have read reports, detailing daily outbursts of temper, where he has variously described the home carers as 'useless fucking bitches' and 'stupid cunts'. He has been reluctant to use the hoist which was installed, and on one occasion pushed the home carer, while she was operating the hoist, with sufficient force to leave bruises. He has criticised the home care service for recruiting 'morons'. The home care manager has said that she is unsure she will be able to maintain the service, given the small number of workers who are still willing to work with Mr Heiberg.

Interview between service user – Martin Heiberg, carer – Martha Heiberg and worker – Geraldine Carter

G: Good morning Mrs Heiberg, thank you for agreeing to see me at such short notice.

Mrs H: Good morning, I'm sorry you've had to come out. I kept telling him if he keeps going on the way he is, no one will come here.

G: Can I talk to your husband?

Mrs H: Yes, but I warn you, he's very agitated.

G: Good morning Mr Heiberg.

Mrs H: It's the lady from social services.

Mr H: Yes I can see who she is. I'm not ga-ga. You're the brains behind this excuse for a service that I've had to put up with.

G: I gather you haven't been very happy with things.

Mr H: You're absolutely right, I'm not. I don't know where you get them from, but they might as well be stacking shelves at Tesco's as far as I'm concerned.

G: There seem to be difficulties on both sides. I'm here to see if there is some way we can resolve them.

Mr H: Well I would suggest getting rid of most of those fucking useless cows you've sent round here.

G: I understand you may not be very happy with the service, but it is not going to get us very far if you continue to describe the staff in such offensive terms. This is part of the reason why some of them are no longer willing to work with you.

Mr H: Well that suits me. I don't want them back anyway. Good riddance to bad rubbish, that's what I say.

G: Well the problem is Mr Heiberg, we might be getting to the point where we don't have enough staff willing to cover the service we are currently putting in.

Mr H: Well that's marvellous, so if I complain, you're just going to leave us, leave my wife to cope on her own.

G: I didn't say that, but I think you do need to understand that there are aspects of your behaviour which have upset some of the carers and made them reluctant to work with you. We don't expect our staff to put up with offensive or abusive insults.

Mr H: So you're saying I've just got to put up with it.

G: The other area of concern is the hoist. I gather that although you were assessed as requiring a hoist, you don't like the staff using it. I believe there was one occasion when a worker was hurt, when you pushed her.

Mr H: That was her stupid fault. She got in the way, didn't know what she was doing. Some of them arrive here not having a clue. Have you seen what they write on those damned sheets they leave here? It's a joke. They're illiterate some of them.

G: Mr Heiberg, if you have specific complaints about the service then I think it's important to discuss them. You have the information about making a formal complaint, and if you feel that you need to do that, then the department will certainly investigate the issues you raise. However, insulting the staff is not going to help, and the hoist is a necessary piece of equipment to ensure your own safety as well as the staff's. You say that you think some of the carers are illiterate and don't know what they're doing. What do you mean?

Mr H: Well they can't spell and what they write, well – it's so pathetic. 'Mr Heiberg did not want his breakfast and seemed angry this morning'. What's the use of that? If I'm angry I'll let people know. And it's a different one every time, so they don't know what they're doing.

G: Well, it is difficult to ensure that the same carers call and, as I've said, part of the problem is that there are fewer staff who are now prepared to come here. But everyone working with you will be working from the care plan, so they should know what they have to do. But, as I say, your behaviour has upset quite a number of people.

Mr H: Well that's a shame. I suppose no one's bothered about me. How do you think I feel stuck in this fucking chair. I don't give a fuck about their feelings.

G: Mr Heiberg, I am trying to help. Your accident was three years ago. You moved into this area three months ago. Did you have problems with the home care service where you previously lived?

Mr H: I suppose there were some problems, but it's much worse here. I never wanted to come here, but it was her, she wanted to be near her bloody family.

Mrs H: I couldn't cope where we used to live. It was all getting too much, you know it was. And my two brothers suggested we move nearer to them so they could help out more.

Mr H: Great fucking help they've been.

Mrs H: Well I'm glad they're nearer. I don't feel so alone anymore.

Mr H: Oh so you're on your own are you? I don't count? I'm not really here. I'm just the pain in the neck you're left looking after.

Mrs H: There's no point talking to you when you're like this. (leaves the room)

Mr H: See, she doesn't want to know.

G: Mr Heiberg you are clearly very angry ..

Mr H: How much do they pay you for that fucking amazing insight?

G: Your anger is making it hard for anyone to help you. It seems as though the move has been difficult for you, and I'm still trying to look at how we can work together to ensure you get the help you need.

Mr H: I didn't want to come here. I knew she'd just be all in with her family again. I never got on with any of them, jumped up nobodies all of them.

G: How much do you think those feelings are influencing your attitude towards the home carers?

Mr H: Maybe, so what?

G: I'm just trying to work out what the problem really is.

Mr H: You're saying I'm the problem?

G: No, I'm saying that you're feeling angry about a number of things, but the target of your anger may not be the actual cause of your anger. I'm thinking particularly of the home carers.

Mr H: So?

G: So maybe it might be helpful for you to talk to someone about those feelings.

Mr H: You mean a fucking counsellor?

G: That could be an option.

Mr H: So if I talk to a counsellor, then I'll learn to be a good boy and behave myself, and stop upsetting those silly cows when they come round.

G: Certainly I don't think it's going to help you or anyone if we get to a stage where no home carer is willing to work here anymore. But as I said if you wish to make a formal complaint then it will be investigated.

Mr H: O.K. you've made your point. I'll think about it. Now if you don't mind there's a radio programme I wanted to hear. Martha, turn the fucking radio on will you?

G: Would it be helpful if I called back in another week, say Friday morning, when you've had time to think about what I've said?

Mr H: Alright, you're persistent, I'll give you that.

G: So I'll see you in a week. Good bye Mr Heiberg.

HO 3a: Suggested record: Transcript: Martin Heiberg

Date of interview: 7.9.04
Worker: Geraldine Carter
Present: Mr Martin Heiberg and Mrs Martha Heiberg
Purpose of visit: To discuss problems in relation to the home care package experienced by the home care service and Mr Heiberg.

I outlined to Mr Heiberg the problem, as it has been described to me by the home care services. Mr Heiberg said that he is dissatisfied with the service, and referred to the home care workers as 'fucking useless cows'. I explained that it was using such offensive language which had led to a number of home carers refusing to work with him, and that there was a danger there would not be enough staff available to cover the current level of service. I also raised the issue of the hoist, and in particular the occasion when a home carer said Mr Heiberg had pushed her, which had resulted in bruising. Mr Heiberg said she had 'got in the way'.

Mr Heiberg continued to criticise the competence of the home care workers, saying they 'haven't a clue' and are 'illiterate'. He also stated that 'it was a different one every time'. I explained the complaints procedure, as well as pointing out that the home care workers work to a care plan, and so should know what to do. I also said that we do try to ensure the same workers call, but part of the problem is that there were fewer home care workers willing to visit.

I asked whether Mr Heiberg had experienced similar problems before he moved to this area, which was three months ago. He said that, although there had been some problems, 'it was much worse here'. He then went on to say that he had never wanted to move to this area, and it was because his wife wanted to live near her family, with whom he had never got on. Mrs Heiberg said she had found it difficult to cope, and needed more help, and now didn't 'feel so alone'.

I suggested to Mr Heiberg that he was very angry, and that anger was making it difficult for anyone to help him. I suggested that his anger about the move might be influencing his attitude to the home carers, and that it might be helpful to talk about those feelings. I restated that it would not help anyone if we got to the stage where no home carer was prepared to work with him. He said he would think about seeing a counsellor. I suggested seeing him in a week, after he has had time to consider my suggestion. It was agreed that I would call on Friday 15 September.

HO 4: Transcript: Fay Goldstein, white Jewish

Fay Goldstein, aged 87, is a widow living on her own in sheltered accommodation. She was diagnosed with Alzheimer's Disease four years ago. She had a fall six years ago, when she broke the bones in three fingers of her right hand. She is right handed, and the subsequent more limited movement of this hand has caused her problems. The left side of her face and neck is badly scarred from a scald she received when she was sixteen. Fay has no children. Her only remaining family is a sister, aged 91, who is living in Israel. They have not communicated for sometime. Fay receives two home care visits a day to help with personal care and meal preparation.

Fay's increasing confusion is causing concern to staff and residents at the sheltered housing complex. Her neighbour complained of the smell of gas on various occasions, and a decision was made to disconnect the gas supply. She has been found walking around the building at night, knocking on people's doors, and has been brought back by the police on at least six occasions, having been found in the road at night in her night clothes. She also tried to give the window cleaner £100 when he last called.

Interview between service user – Fay Goldstein and worker – Ben Napley

B: Good morning Mrs Goldstein.
FG: Hello dear, you're early, I wasn't expecting you till this evening,
B: I did telephone to say I would call this morning.
FG: Did you dear, oh I'm sorry, if I'd known I would have got something nice.
B: Don't worry about that Mrs Goldstein. I have come to see how you are.
FG: Oh that is kind, well I've been very busy you know, I've just come back from the Far East, it was a long way you know.
B: I'm not sure that you've been abroad recently.
FG: I picked up this bug you know, you get those sort of things out there, stomach upsets, not very nice really. I wouldn't like you to catch it.
B: I'm sure I'll be alright. Are you feeling unwell then?
FG: Well I said to someone that I thought I had picked something up, but I don't think I've got a temperature. It was that fall probably. I fell out of bed you know.
B: How did you do that?
FG: I don't know. Somebody keeps moving everything around in here, they keep leaving their rubbish.
(Door bell rings)
FG: Well I wonder who that could be? (goes to the door)
Josie (warden): Hello, Mrs Goldstein, how are you this morning? Oh I can see you have a visitor. I won't disturb you. Everything alright?
FG: Well I said to this nice gentleman that I don't think I'm quite myself.
J: Why's that then?
FG: Well I don't know really.
B: Mrs Goldstein said she had a fall.
J: That was over a week ago and it wasn't really a fall was it? You tripped when you went into the lounge downstairs and knocked a lamp over. It didn't break though, but it did shake you up a bit.

FG: Oh dear, I'm glad I didn't break anything.

J: I'll leave you to carry on talking to Ben.

FG: Oh thank you, (closes door, turns to Ben) Can I get you anything?

B: No, that's very kind. I just wanted to talk about how you were, and if there was anything more we could do to help.

FG: Well that's very sweet of you.

B: Mrs Goldstein, I gather you have been going out at night, and the police have brought you back on a number of occasions.

FG: Yes, I needed to go to the shops.

B: But the shops won't be open at night.

FG: Oh, they're very good round here, it's so handy when you find you've just run out of something. I'm always doing that. I get through so much milk. It's next door you know. They come and take it. I mean I don't mind, but I wish they'd ask. They're always having parties. They're having one now. Can't you hear them? (no sound).

B: I can't actually hear anything Mrs Goldstein.

FG: Oh yes, they're having a high old time.

B: How do you think you are managing?

FG: I musn't grumble really.

B: Do you think you could do with more help?

FG: Mummy used to have help you know, for the heavy work, she was never strong really.

B: How do you get on with the people here?

FG: I just wish they'd be quieter. Do you want a cup of tea? I'm going to have one. (Gets up and puts a tea bag in a mug and fills it with water from the hot tap)

B: No, it's alright thank you. Mrs Goldstein, I am concerned that you seem quite confused this morning.

FG: Do I dear? Well when you get to my age you know.

B: I am just wondering how you might feel about living somewhere where people can look after you more. You only have the home carers coming in twice a day, and I wonder whether that is enough. I am particularly worried about you going out at night.

FG: Well I should really like to go back to Chiswick. I used to have a very nice house there after the war.

B: I'm sorry, I won't be able to arrange that, but it might be that we could find somewhere where you would be more safe. I could take you to see a very nice home, and you could think about whether you would like to live there.

FG: Well, that is kind but I'm very busy.

B: Well let me go away and think about what we could offer, and I'll call back in a little while.

FG: Alright then dear, so nice of you to call.

HO 4a: Suggested record: Transcript: Fay Goldstein

Date of interview: 29.11.03
Worker: Ben Napley
Present: Mrs Fay Goldstein
Purpose of visit: To monitor care package in response to concerns raised by staff from Kelso Lodge, the sheltered housing complex where Mrs Goldstein lives.

During my visit Mrs Goldstein appeared rather confused. She stated she had just returned from the Far East and had picked up a bug. She then thought the bug may have been caused by falling out of bed. I asked what had happened and she said that somebody keeps moving things around in her flat and that they leave rubbish.

Mrs Robinson, the warden called during my visit and explained that the fall to which Mrs Goldstein had referred, happened over a week ago when Mrs Goldstein had knocked over a lamp in the communal lounge.

I raised the issue with Mrs Goldstein about her going out at night and being brought back by the police. She said she needed to go out to the shops, despite my pointing out they would be closed. She said she needed to get milk because her neighbours come and take it. She also said they were always having parties and believed there was one going on while I was there. I said I couldn't hear anything. While I was there I observed Mrs Goldstein making tea with hot water from the tap.

I asked how she thought she was managing, and whether she might want some more help. Mrs Goldstein then went on to talk about her mother needing help 'with the heavy work'. I observed that she seemed confused. She then connected her confusion with her age. I asked her whether she might like to live 'somewhere where people can look after you more'. She said she would like to go back to her house in Chiswick that she lived in after the war. I suggested taking her to see a home, where she could be more safe, and that she could think about whether she might like to live there. She said she was very busy. I said I would call back to see her in a little while.

Trainer's notes

(The worker would need to go on and discuss the significance of this conversation with Mrs Goldstein in terms of what it suggests about her current level of confusion. It is important however to have on record an accurate description of what a service user is saying and what they are doing, in order to understand the extent of the problem. Even when the behaviour may appear irrational, it is still important to describe that behaviour, so that the reader has an objective account from which they can reach their own judgement.)

▣ HO 5: Transcript: Vincent Morris, white

Vincent Morris, aged 61, and Nicholas Baird, aged 50, have lived together for fifteen years as a couple. Vincent was diagnosed with Motor Neurone disease five years ago. He now uses a wheelchair and has some movement in his arms and hands. He is able to feed himself, but needs help with washing, dressing and using the toilet. His partner Nicholas works full-time as a commissioning editor with a publishing company. Vincent also used to work in publishing.

Vincent has one home care visit in the morning to help get him up, prepare his breakfast and leave his lunch. Nicholas leaves at 6.00 am to travel to London daily. He arrives home at 7.00 pm, prepares the evening meal, and helps Vincent get ready for bed. Vincent has called the office to say Nicholas has to go to America in a month for a conference, and will then be staying on to see friends. Vincent will need additional help for the two weeks Nicholas is away. You read that Vincent said he 'was dreading Nicholas going' when he phoned the office. You are visiting to identify what further help Vincent will need while Nicholas is away.

Interview between service user – Vincent Morris and worker – Lucy Stratford

L: Good morning, Vincent.

V: Hello.

L: How are you?

V: Not very good really.

L: I heard you were not very happy about Nicholas going away.

V: Yes I really don't want to be on my own for that long.

L: Well I thought it would be useful to talk about how we could help you while he is away. When is he going?

V: In a month, he flies out on the 21st.

L: And it's for two weeks.

V: Yes, he only needs to go for four days, but he wants to stay longer to see some friends.

L: And how do you feel about that?

V: Well I can't stop him can I? And he needs a break. I know he finds it difficult. I suppose I should count myself lucky he's stayed with me this long.

L: What do you mean?

V: Well, he's a lot younger than me anyway. What's he got to look forward to sticking with me? Why should he carry on looking after me until the end, when he's just going to be left getting older alone?

L: Have you talked with him about this?

V: Not really, I mean, what can you say. It's not something either of us ever thought about. Nicholas has been very good. He's always patient, puts up with my moods, but you know the relationship changes when you become so dependent on someone.

L: Would you prefer it if Nicholas wasn't so involved in your personal care?

V: I'd prefer it if I didn't need anyone to look after me, but, yes, I do find it more difficult with Nicholas. You know it's strange really, he's so much more involved with me in all the physical care, and yet I think we are further apart emotionally than ever.

L: Do you find it difficult to talk?

V: Yes I think there is so much we try and avoid, because we just don't know what to say, and I'm just scared he's going to leave me, I mean I wouldn't blame him if he did, but I don't know what I'd do. Well there wouldn't be any point anymore?

L: What do you mean?

V: Well Nicholas is the only reason I keep going on. If I didn't have him, there would be no point in carrying on with all this. The only trouble is I'm not sure I could do anything about it now without someone's help.

L: You're talking about someone helping you to die?

V: Yes, if Nicholas wasn't here then I wouldn't want to go on anymore, I mean why on earth would I?

L: You seem to have become very anxious about Nicholas. You've been together a long time. Why do you think he might not stay with you?

V: Ever since I got the diagnosis I've wondered how long he would stay. And I suppose after five years you might think he's not going to go now. But, like I said, it's harder to talk and I know it's all getting too much for him, which is why he wants to get away, so he can decide what he really wants now.

L: Nicholas may simply need a break. That doesn't mean he's thinking of anything beyond that. Would it help if I talked to him?

V: No, I don't want you to say anything about any of this to him. It would only make him feel more trapped.

L: I do think it would help to share some of this with him. It seems as though you are putting up barriers between you which are making things worse.

V: No, I can't talk about this with him. I can't beg him to stay. I want him to stay, but only if he wants to. No he's got to sort that out for himself.

L: But you may be worrying about this trip to America for nothing. I'm not sure it's going to be a good idea for you to be on your own while Nicholas is away. I had thought we might increase the home care for the two weeks, but I'm wondering if you might be better going in to stay at somewhere like Wessex Lodge, on a respite basis.

V: I don't know about that. I like my own space. I'm not sure what would be worse, having to fit in with a load of strangers for two weeks, or be on my own.

L: Are there any friends or family who could come and stay during that time?

V: No, Nicholas and I don't have any family now, and we don't see, well I don't see much of our friends anymore.

L: What do you mean?

V: Well I know Nicholas still sees some of them, but they don't come to the house anymore. They can't face me.

L: I am concerned at how you are feeling today Vincent.

V: Well wouldn't you feel the same if you were in my position?

L: I don't know, but I would like to try and help. I am not sure that increasing the home care to two or even three visits a day while Nicholas is away is necessarily the right answer. I would like you to think about Wessex Lodge. I could always take you to visit beforehand, so you could see what it is like. And I also think it might help for you to try and talk with Nicholas, or perhaps you might benefit from outside help in talking about your situation.

V: I'm not sure about that. I'd rather stay in my own home, and if you just arrange for someone to come round in the evening as well as the morning, then that will probably be enough. Nicholas will leave me some frozen meals so I just need help getting to bed. The rest I'll have to manage and hope Nicholas and I can sort things out between us.

L: Well I wonder, going back to what you were saying earlier about the effect on your relationship of Nicholas being involved with your personal care. Perhaps it might help to increase the home care input even after Nicholas comes back.

V: Yes, that is something that might help. I don't know. I'd like to think about that and that's something I could talk to Nicholas about, although I would have to be careful and not make him feel I was rejecting him. Can you give me time to think about that. If you don't mind I'm feeling quite tired now. Could we finish? I think we've covered everything.

L: Yes, of course. I'll arrange for Home Care to be increased to two visits a day while Nicholas is away, but if there is anything else I can help you with, do ring me.

V: Thank you, you've been very kind.

L: Well, bye for now.

HO 5a: Suggested record: Transcript: Vincent Morris

Date of interview: 18.7.04
Worker: Lucy Stratford
Present: Vincent Morris
Purpose of visit: To assess needs for two weeks while carer is away.

Vincent Morris explained that his partner and carer, Nicholas Baird will be attending a conference in America, flying out on the 21 August. He will then be spending a further two weeks visiting friends. Vincent says he is not happy at the prospect of being on his own for that time. Vincent acknowledged that Nicholas needed a break, but he was worried that Nicholas's role as a carer has changed their relationship. Vincent said that even though Nicholas was more involved in Vincent's physical care, Vincent felt they were further apart emotionally. He said he felt there was so much they found difficult to talk about. Vincent said he was scared Nicholas would leave him. He feels that Nicholas has looked after him for five years, but it may be 'all getting too much for him' and Nicholas is using the trip to get away and decide what he really wants. Vincent feels that, as Nicholas is a lot younger than him, he has little to look forward to staying with Vincent.

Vincent said that, without Nicholas, he would see no point in going on, but said he didn't think he could do anything about it without someone's help. I asked if he meant wanting someone to help to die, and he repeated that without Nicholas he would not want to continue living.

I suggested that Nicholas may simply need a break, without that meaning that he is thinking of leaving. I asked if it would help if I talked to Nicholas. Vincent said he did not want Nicholas to know anything of what had been discussed between us concerning their relationship.

I suggested that given Vincent's anxieties, and as he said he had no family and saw little of friends, it might not be a good idea for him to be on his own for two weeks, and that perhaps he might like to consider Wessex Lodge on a respite basis. Vincent said he liked his 'own space', and didn't like the idea of having 'to fit in with strangers'. Vincent said he preferred having an extra home care call in the evening to help put him to bed. Nicholas would leave a stock of frozen meals, so he would not need any help with food.

I suggested that Vincent might want to think about the home care input being increased on a permanent basis. This would mean that Nicholas did not have to be so involved in Vincent's personal care. Vincent thought that might help, and would discuss it with Nicholas, although he was concerned not to make Nicholas feel he was being rejected. He wanted time to think about the idea. It was agreed that for the two weeks Nicholas is away, Home Care calls will be increased to two visits daily, to include a putting to bed call.

Section C: 'A medical opinion is a fact'

This quote from a course participant illustrates some of the complexity around this issue. Many workers will simply see this in terms of the need to include 'In my opinion' before any statement, where they feel they have expressed a judgement. This ignores the very basic way in which the language we use to describe situations can itself reflect our attitudes and opinions about that situation.

There is also a feeling that resorting to the terms 'it seemed' or 'it appeared' provides at least an acknowledgement that this is how the situation appeared to me, but it might not be the same for someone else. This goes some way to address the problem, but there are still questions which may be left unanswered. What behaviour or what did someone say which led the worker to think that someone 'seemed anxious'? This is quite separate from any speculation about the possible reasons why they might be anxious. It is concerned with what the objective evidence was which led to the conclusion that someone seemed anxious.

This section will require the trainer to introduce the topic with some information before going on to the exercises.

✔ Exercise 4: What is fact and what is opinion?

↗ Objective

To explore the distinction between fact and opinion

🕐 Timing

Allow 30 minutes for this exercise

✏ Materials

- HO 6: Distinguishing fact and opinion
- HO 7: What is fact and what is opinion?
- Pens and paper
- Overhead projector
- OHT 1: Distinguishing fact and opinion

ⓘ Trainer's guidelines

Step 1: allow 15 minutes
Introduce OHT1. Allow participants the opportunity to respond to the points. Make links between the issues around fact and opinion with the issues raised in the introduction to the chapter, looking at the problem of selective perception.

Give out HO 6: Distinguishing fact and opinion

Step 2: allow 15 minutes
This exercise can be done in small groups, but it works just as effectively with a whole group.

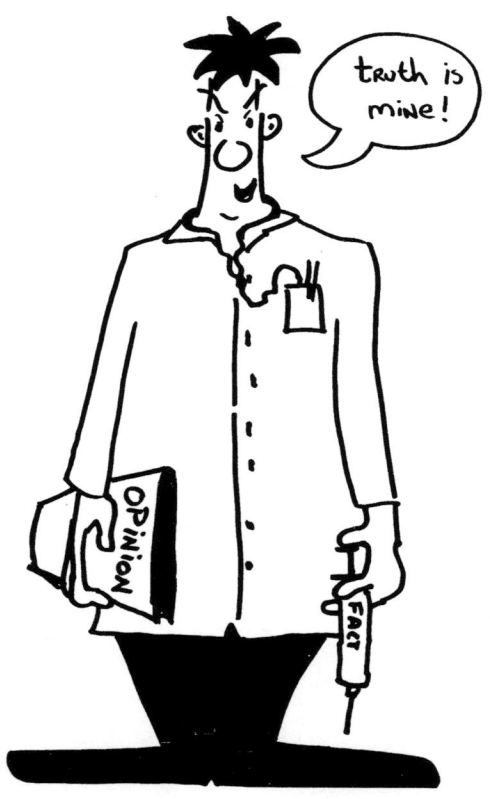

Give out HO 7: What is fact and what is opinion?

Read out each statement in turn and ask participants to call out whether they think a statement is fact or opinion.

Refer to answer sheet for further guidance.

OHT 1: Distinguishing fact and opinion

- # Be clear about the status of information

  o Verifiable factual information

  o Direct observations

  o Understandings

  o Hearsay

  o Opinions, judgements, evaluations, recommendations

- # Beware the adjective

- # Beware opinions masquerading as facts

  o Reinforced or shared opinion

  o Expert opinion

HO 6: Distinguishing fact and opinion

Be clear about the status of information

- **Verifiable factual information**, this is information that cannot be disputed, hard facts, e.g. dates of birth, who attended a meeting.
- **Direct observations** by the worker. Observations are sometimes difficult to locate in terms of the hierarchy of fact through to opinion. If the worker observes someone feeding themselves without assistance or records that someone has said, 'I feel exhausted', these are factual statements. However, some observations can involve subjective interpretation and so may move closer to opinion. This is particularly relevant where the same situation could be viewed differently by the various people present.
- **Understandings** are statements about how things appear, that are assumed to be true, but should not be considered as facts, e.g. 'It seemed that', 'It appeared that'. This at least acknowledges that this is how a situation appeared to that particular worker, but there are still questions which may be left unanswered. What behaviour or conversation led the worker to think that someone 'seemed anxious'? What was the objective evidence which led to the conclusion that someone seemed anxious?
- **Hearsay** is an account given by someone else and is therefore unsubstantiated, second-hand information and should not be considered as fact. The source of the information should be clearly identified.
- **Opinions, judgements, evaluations, recommendations** may be based on a collective view, a considered review by the worker or agreed with the service user. This forms an important part of social care work, although the basis and reason for the opinion should also be stated with reference to supporting information.

Beware of the adjective

We need to be aware of how we can often suggest a factual account, which is actually opinion, simply by the way we use language in our record. For instance if we describe someone as being either optimistic or pessimistic, they are both statements of opinion. Using an adjective without any evidence or explanation as to why we think that adjective is appropriate, is a limited and unhelpful statement of opinion.

Beware of opinions masquerading as facts

- **Reinforced or shared opinion.** This often occurs when an opinion is shared by more than one professional, reinforcing that opinion so that it becomes accepted as fact. Instead of being seen as an opinion that is shared by most people, whether that is as a result of convincing or persuasive argument or evidence, the opinion becomes elevated or transformed into a fact. This can also happen in the life of a file, where a view taken by a worker early on in a case, may influence the way in which every subsequent worker approaches that service user.

● **Expert opinion.** This is where the opinion is expressed by someone of such eminence or expert status that their opinion somehow seems beyond question and becomes accepted as fact. So a medical opinion or a diagnosis may be accepted as fact, whereas it is an opinion based on the interpretation of factual evidence, e.g. results of blood tests, observed signs and symptoms.

HO 7: What is fact and what is opinion?

Decide in your groups whether the following statements are fact or opinion.

1. The relationship between Mr and Mrs T has become increasingly strained.
2. Mrs F is incapable of handling her finances.
3. Mrs O complained that her home carer was late yesterday.
4. Mr J lacks insight into his wife's condition.
5. The flat is uninhabitable.
6. The injury to Mr K's arm is consistent with being pulled or dragged.
7. This is the first incident of abuse to this lady.
8. I observed Mr V going up and coming down the stairs unaided.
9. Mr G is a resilient and determined man, who displays great fortitude in very difficult circumstances.
10. Mrs W appeared very anxious when I asked her about her neighbour.
11. Dr Foley has said that Mrs N will not be able to manage on her own at home without substantial support.
12. Mr C said he was certain that his daughter had taken his pension book.
13. Mrs J said she was in such pain that she did not want to live anymore.
14. Without additional support Mr Y will be at serious risk.
15. Mrs M was unwilling to discuss her incontinence problems.
16. Mr A has a good relationship with his daughter.
17. Mrs D's family are not supportive.
18. Mr S has become emotionally over dependent on his home carer.
19. Mrs B's daughter was present when I visited and said that she had found soiled clothes in her mother's wardrobe.
20. Mrs P is making considerable progress.

Trainer notes: What is fact and what is opinion?

1. Opinion.
2. Opinion, except if this statement is being made as a result of an individual being legally defined as incapable.
3. Fact – that the statement had been made, although we do not know if it is true, so the content needs to be treated as hearsay.
4. Opinion.
5. Opinion, except if this statement is being made as a result of a dwelling being legally defined as uninhabitable, e.g. If it does not have a roof.
6. Opinion.
7. Opinion. This should more correctly read as 'the first known or recorded incident'.
8. Fact.
9. Opinion.
10. Opinion, how was Mrs W behaving which made her appear anxious?
11. Fact – that Dr Foley said Mrs N will not be able to manage, but Dr Foley is expressing an opinion.
12. Fact – that the statement had been made, although we do not know if it is true, so the content needs to be treated as hearsay
13. Fact.
14. Opinion.
15. Opinion. What did Mrs M say or do which led the worker to conclude she was reluctant to discuss her incontinence problems? Did she ignore the question, maybe she didn't hear it? Did she change the subject? Did she say she didn't want to talk about it? A description of her actual behaviour would be a more objective record of her reaction.
16. Opinion.
17. Opinion.
18. Opinion.
19. Fact – that the statement had been made, although we do not know if it is true, so the content needs to be treated as hearsay.
20. Opinion.

Exercise 5: Being positively objective

Objective

To illustrate the power of language in influencing the way we perceive people and the way in which our accounts can influence colleagues.

Timing

Allow 30 minutes for this exercise

Materials

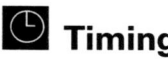

- HO 8: Archie Fenman: older people, or HO 9: Oscar Reynolds: mental health, or HO 10: Joy Fraser: learning disability

Trainer's guidelines

Step 1: allow 5 minutes
Introduce the exercise and divide participants into groups of two, three or four individuals. Give them a copy of the relevant case sheet. Ask them to identify what is fact and what is opinion and to distinguish the status of different information in Versions A and B. Ask them to compare the two versions in terms of how effective they are as sources of information about the individuals described.

Step 2: allow 15 minutes
Participants complete the exercise

Step 3: allow 10 minutes
Ask each group to summarise their discussion, asking them to distinguish fact and opinion and to distinguish the status of different information in Versions A and B. Go on to discuss how effective Versions A and B are as sources of information about the individuals described.

HO 8: Archie Fenman: older people

Version A

Archie Fenman is a 66-year-old white man who lives on his own in a council flat. His wife died four years ago. He was diagnosed with diabetes ten years ago and with cirrhosis of the liver seven years ago. His daughter, Amanda, a single parent who works full-time, lives five miles away and tries to visit once a week. She says she is very worried about her father's drinking. She believes that he drinks two or three bottles of whiskey a week as well as a large quantity of beer. She thinks that he does not eat properly and spends most of his money on drink. She feels he can't be bothered to do anything but drink.

Archie's GP, Dr Raine has said that Archie is at risk and will be dead in two years if he doesn't stop drinking.

When visiting Archie at home, I observed what looked like large amounts of rubbish piled up in each of the rooms. The kitchen was full of unwashed dishes and cartons, many with stale food and bottles. I observed maggots on the stale food and evidence of mice droppings on the floor and kitchen surfaces.

Archie said to me that he didn't care what people thought about him or the way he lived. He said that 'was his business' and he didn't 'want a lot of do-gooders telling him what to do'. He knew his daughter was worried about him but he said she ought to stop interfering.

Archie said that he had been in the merchant navy for most of his working life and he had never wanted to give it up, but when he was 50 his wife had given him an ultimatum, so he reluctantly took a job in a warehouse.

When asked about his drinking and its impact on his health, he said that he didn't care. He knew what the doctor had said. Archie said it wouldn't make any difference now as his 'liver was fucked anyway'. He liked drinking and 'life wouldn't be worth living if he couldn't have a drink'. He said there was nothing else left for him.

Version B

Archie Fenman, aged 66 is an alcoholic with diabetes and cirrhosis of the liver. His doctor has given him two years to live if he doesn't stop drinking. He lives alone in council accommodation. His wife died four years ago. His daughter Amanda, who lives nearby, visits once a week but has failed to persuade her father to stop drinking.

Mr Fenman lives in filthy conditions, has little insight into his condition and is unwilling to do anything to help himself. He is contemptuous of all offers of help.

HO 9: Oscar Reynolds: mental health

Version A

Oscar Reynolds is a 42-year-old, Black Caribbean man, who was born in Wolverhampton five years after his parents emigrated from Jamaica. According to his records, and from Oscar's own account of his life, his sister, who was three years younger than him, died after being knocked down by a car when she was four. Oscar's mother then experienced recurring bouts of depression over the next twelve years. Oscar's father worked on the railways and, because of his shift-work, Oscar lived with his mother's sister when his mum was in hospital. Oscar's aunt belonged to an evangelical church and, according to Oscar, believed in strict discipline. He says that she used to regularly beat him with a strap for what she called his 'badness'. He remembers his aunt blaming his mum for not being firm enough with him.

Oscar says that he never liked school, and that, whenever there was any trouble, he always got the blame, even though he claims the other kids picked on him because he was black. After a fight, where he says the other boy slipped and hit his head against a wall, Oscar was expelled at the age of 13. Oscar says he was never allowed to return to school, and spent most of his time in his room at home. He tried to get a job, after his father threatened to throw him out, but he could never work anywhere more than a few weeks. Oscar says that he found it difficult to get on with people, and remembers someone telling him he was insubordinate, although he never knew what that meant.

According to the record and Oscar's own account, at the age of 16 Oscar came home to find his mother lying in the bath after cutting her wrists. He called for help from the neighbours and she was rushed to hospital. She survived, although she told Oscar she wished he had let her die. Oscar said he can't remember much about what happened after this, but he was arrested after breaking into a mortuary and cutting up the bodies he found there with a meat cleaver. According to his records he was diagnosed with schizophrenia and sent to a secure mental hospital. He did not want to talk about his time in hospital except to say that he 'learnt to be good'.

He was released from hospital after 20 years and returned to live with his widowed mother. Oscar says he was unable to work, and his mother helped to support him. Oscar says that it was after he came home that he started to put on a lot of weight. He is 6 ft 6 ins tall and presently weighs 30 stone. During this time he says he liked to play music, and spent most of his time in the house.

Six months ago Oscar's mother died of a heart attack, and since then his behaviour has been causing concern to his family and neighbours. He has accused his relatives of poisoning his mother. He remembers her saying before she died, 'I've been poisoned'. His aunt claims that she has seen him standing outside their house, staring at her, and that she is frightened of him. Neighbours are complaining that the house has become very dirty and neglected. The garden is full of rubbish and attracting rats. Oscar says that people throw rubbish into his garden, and that he just feels tired all the time and can't cope with the house. The neighbours have phoned social services, saying they can see Oscar in the garden talking and shouting to himself. Oscar says that he thinks his aunt and her family are trying to kill him.

Version B

Oscar Reynolds is a 42-year-old Black Caribbean man, who was diagnosed with schizophrenia at the age of 17, following an incident where he broke into a mortuary and proceeded to butcher the bodies he found there with a meat cleaver. He then spent 20 years in a secure mental hospital.

Oscar had a troubled school history. He was seen as aggressive and violent and was expelled at the age of 13. He did not finish his education. He has failed to work even when not in hospital and relied on his mother to support him. She has a history of depression and has attempted suicide.

Since her death six months ago, his behaviour has become more unpredictable and disturbed. His family are frightened of him and his neighbours feel he is a menace and living in squalid conditions. He is grossly obese.

HO 10: Joy Fraser: learning disability

Version A

Joy Fraser is a 22-year-old white woman who has a mild learning disability and lives at home with her mother and step-father and two brothers in Glasgow. Joy attends a local day centre, where she has established a number of positive relationships with other service users. At a social event Joy met Gus King, who she describes as her boy-friend. Gus works in a local warehouse and lives in a supported group home with two other people, with staff support for two hours each day. Joy says she wants to live with Gus and 'have babies'.

Joy's mother is very anxious about the relationship between Gus and Joy, saying that she feels Joy is not capable of living independently. Mrs Fraser describes herself as devout Catholic and believes that Joy is at risk of being 'taken advantage of' in her relationship with Gus. She believes that Joy is 'very innocent' and fears that Joy will become pregnant. Mrs Fraser has opposed Joy receiving any contraceptive advice, believing this is contrary to the teachings of the church. She describes Joy as always wanting babies 'without understanding where they come from'. She says that Joy played with her dolls until she was eighteen as though they were real babies and used to 'get cross if people did not go along with her'.

Mrs Fraser said that she is under a lot of strain at the moment as her youngest son, aged 9, who is the only child of her second marriage, has been truanting from school, saying he is being bullied. She says her husband works away a lot, and she feels she is left to manage on her own. Joy's father died when she was 10 years old.

Joy has said that she wants to live with Gus, but does not want her mother to know this. When it has been pointed out that her mother will need to know if she is going to leave her family home, she says that she doesn't want to tell her mother and that she just wants to go. She says that her mother will try to stop her. She says that once she is living with Gus, 'he will look after her.'

Version B

Joy Fraser is 22-years-old and has a mild learning disability. She lives at home and attends a day centre. She wants to live with her boy-friend Gus King, who also has a learning disability. Her mother is opposed to this and is worried about Joy becoming pregnant, despite not wanting Joy to receive contraceptive advice.

Chapter 2: We Know Just What You Need

Section A: Introduction – problems with assessments

Assessments are central to the work of social service departments. They are the primary task of social workers and care managers working in adult services. Practitioners believe they work with the best interests of the service user in mind. So why do the records of assessments continue to be criticised for being:

- Service led rather than needs led?
- Not holistic or balanced, with too much emphasis on weaknesses and deficits?
- Not focused on outcomes?

There may be a number of organisational factors which influence the way practitioners approach their task.

Service led rather than needs led

Everyone develops a routinised way of working to some extent. When we are engaged in similar tasks on a regular basis, we develop an expertise based on accumulated experience. That experience may lead us to see work in terms of familiar categories. We've seen a certain kind of situation before and we recognise the same characteristics in a new situation, and so it is natural to develop certain patterns of response. 'Oh that's a so-and-so situation, and this is what we usually do.'

However, when this is applied to assessments in social care, it can easily lead to the service led approach. Most people will disassociate themselves from this,

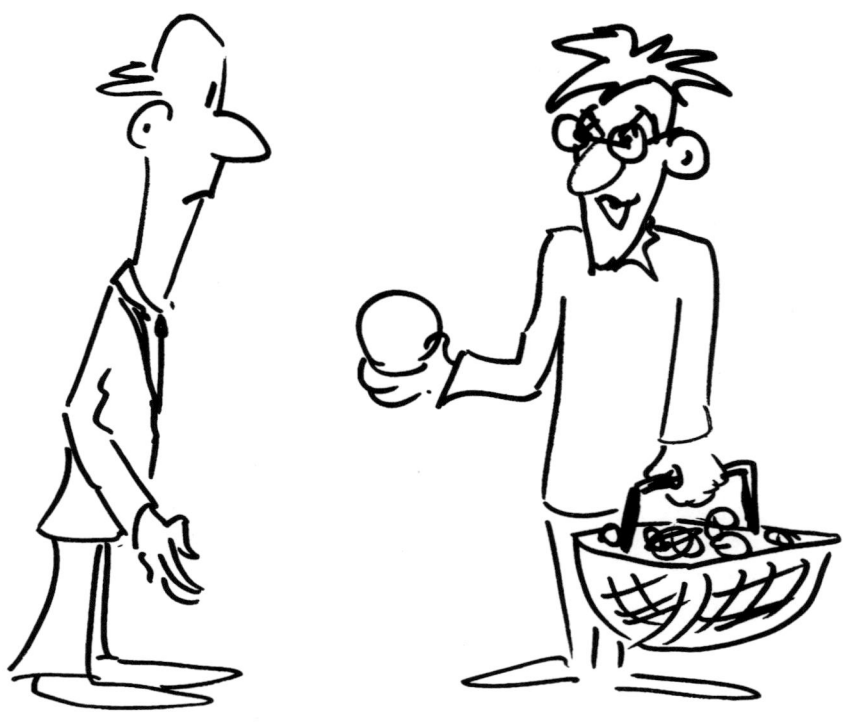

but when you start exploring how they actually work, it is interesting how readily the service led response is adopted. In exercises which are designed to ask participants to identify a service user's needs, there is a strong tendency to immediately start talking about the sort of service which will be most appropriate or effective to meet the needs, before the needs have even been properly defined. This may occur because of pressure on time, or it might be the worker's concern to provide help and support, to get the services in, and do something to help the service user.

Not holistic or balanced, emphasising deficits and weaknesses

Again there are real dilemmas facing many practitioners. Many believe that unless they describe the service user in the most needy terms, they will not make a sufficiently effective case for the resources they believe the service user requires. There is a perception that, if strengths are highlighted, this will make the individual's case weaker in terms of the eligibility criteria. Practitioners have said on training courses that they sometimes feel the need to warn their service users that they will not recognise themselves in their assessments.

Not focused on outcomes

Practitioners will often complain that writing outcome objectives feels very much like trying to rewrite the needs. The exercise may involve little more than simply finding a different form of words. Many practitioners struggle with this task, and resent what they see as time-wasting administration for its own sake. Few seem to have had very clear guidance on what an outcome objective might look like.

Each of these issues is addressed in this chapter, but before we go any further it may be useful to first explore the way in which the assessment interview is experienced by both the practitioner and the service user.

Exercise 6: Seeing the whole picture

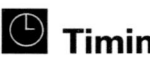 **Objective**

To reflect on the interview process, both from the perspective of the service user and the practitioner.

🕐 **Timing**

Allow 55 minutes for this exercise

✏️ **Materials**

- Flipchart and marker pens
- Pens and paper
- HO 11a and HO 11b: Billy Ellis, or HO 12a and HO 12b: Terry Jakes

ⓘ **Trainer's guidelines**

Step 1: allow 10 minutes
Introduce the exercise. Divide the group into pairs. In the event of an odd number, one group will need to include an observer. Ask each pair to decide who will take the role of the care manager, and who will take the role of the service user. Give out the HOs, 'a' to the 'service user' and 'b' to the 'care manager'. Explain that the 'service user' has more detailed information than the 'care manager'. The 'service user' can decide how much information they will share with the care manager during the interview, but they must not show the 'care manager' their case sheet. The 'service user' will need a few minutes to familiarise themselves with their character and situation. The 'care manager' is asked to find out the 'service user's' needs in the time available for the interview.

Step 2: allow 15 minutes
Allow the pairs to role play their assessment interviews. Give warning when the interviews have two minutes left.

Step 3: allow 15 minutes
Bring the group back together and review the role play. Explain that the 'service users' may have varied in the way they were played, some will have been more emotional than others. Ask the 'care managers' to describe very briefly what sort of 'service user' they interviewed. Reassure the 'service users' that they will have their turn a little later. Go on to ask the 'care managers' in turn to identify one of the 'service user's' needs. Keep going round the group of 'care managers' until all the needs are listed. Note whether needs or services are being identified.

Step 4: allow 15 minutes
Now ask the 'service users' to comment on the list of needs. How far do they feel it reflects what they saw as their needs? Ask them to comment on how it felt listening to the previous discussion of their needs. It is interesting that there is usually a variation between those 'service users' who appreciated the opportunity to talk about how they felt, and those who were looking for the practitioner to provide solutions to their problems. Conclude the exercise with

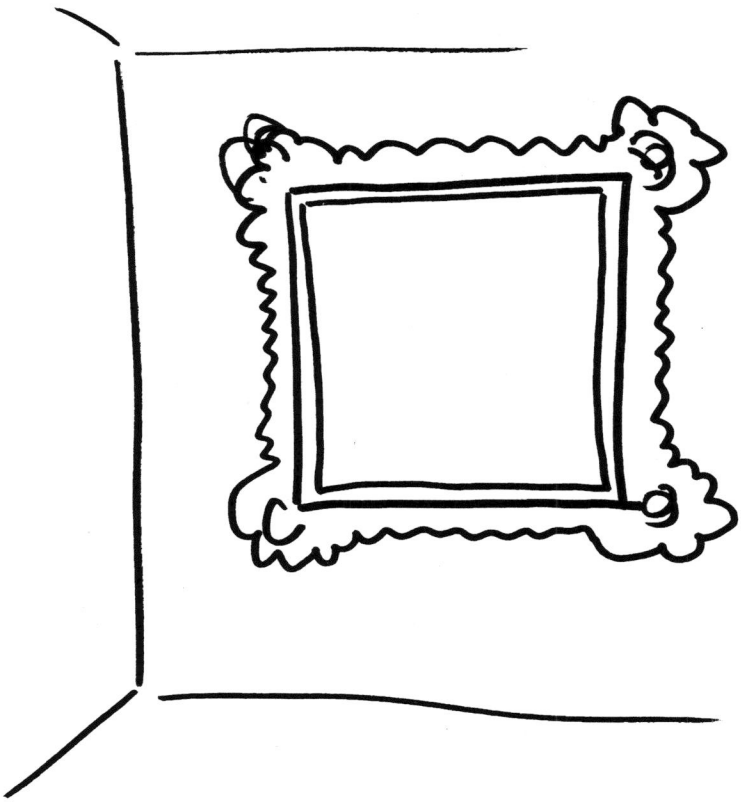

an acknowledgement that the exercise was demanding for both parties in the role play. The 'care manager' had the pressure of trying to find out what were the 'service user's' actual needs and at the same time demonstrate empathic listening. The 'service users' were required to take on the role of someone in very distressing circumstances, and they may need the opportunity to de-role. This can be incorporated into the general discussion at the end of the exercise. Any individuals who appear to need further support should be seen separately.

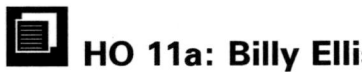 **HO 11a: Billy Ellis**

Service user: Briefing sheet

Billy Ellis is a 35-year-old, mature student, in the second year of a degree course studying sociology. Billy has been having problems with his sight for sometime; glasses have not been able to help. Billy has also been feeling extremely tired, with very painful sensations in his arms, hands and legs. His balance has become more difficult. At first Billy put it down to the demands of studying as well as the problems he was experiencing in his relationship. Billy felt his partner didn't understand why he wanted to do the degree, and resented the financial sacrifices involved. Billy had previously had a reasonably well paid job as a chef, but wanted to do something that was going to be more meaningful and hoped to go into teaching. Now Billy's partner has met someone else, but isn't sure whether the relationship with Billy is really over. They have no children and the house is in his partner's name. Billy moved in after his partner's first marriage ended.

Billy has recently been diagnosed with Multiple Sclerosis. He has found the news very frightening, as the only people he knows about who have had the disease have ended up in wheelchairs, become very ill and died young. Billy is now feeling extremely depressed and finding it more difficult to cope with his course. Billy has thought about suicide and mentioned this to his doctor, who has put Billy on anti-depressants. Billy feels these have just made him feel more ill.

Billy feels he is in danger of losing everything that is important to him, and feels helpless to do anything about it.

HO 11b: Care manager: Briefing sheet

Billy Ellis is a 35-year-old, mature student, who has been diagnosed with Multiple Sclerosis. He has considerable problems with his vision which is making it difficult to study. Billy Ellis has been referred by his GP for support.

HO 12a: Terry Jakes

Service user: Briefing sheet

Terry Jakes is 50-years-old and has lived on benefit for the last 15 years, after serving a prison sentence of two years for an assault against his partner. Terry stabbed his partner in the stomach; the partner then spent two months in hospital recovering from her wounds. Terry's defence was that his partner was unfaithful and also violent. Terry felt the assault happened because he was driven to breaking point and could not cope anymore. Terry said he was still in love with his partner and could not leave her. Terry was diagnosed with depression in his early 20s and has had recurrent bouts throughout his adult life.

Terry's parents died in a car accident when he was 12 and he was subsequently fostered, although all three placements broke down. Terry then lived in residential care from the age of 15 to 18 and subsequently moved from this area.

Terry has lived alone in a privately rented room since coming out of prison, and lost all contact with his former partner. There was one child from the relationship, who Terry has also not seen since the assault. Terry has developed a drink problem, and also smokes heavily. Both have taken a toll on his health.

Terry spends his time listening to the radio, and still occasionally plays the piano. Terry used to be a professional musician. Terry also continues to write short stories, but has never tried to get them published.

Terry has just been made homeless after a fire in his room. Terry's landlord is refusing to have him back, believing the fire was started by one of Terry's cigarette stubs. Terry was injured and is now recovering in hospital. The doctor has advised that Terry's right hand and arm, which were badly burned, will take a long time to heal and feels that Terry will need support after discharge.

HO 12b: Care manager: Briefing sheet

Terry Jakes is 50-years-old and living on benefit. He has a history of alcohol problems and has been in prison for stabbing his partner 17 years ago. He is now in hospital after a fire in his room. His landlord is refusing to allow Terry to return, believing Terry carelessly started the fire. Terry has severely burned his right hand and arm and the doctor is advising Terry will require support after discharge.

Section B: Whose need is it anyway?

 Exercise 7: Identifying needs

Objective

To develop a needs led approach to assessment, which is holistic and non-prescriptive.

Timing

Allow 2 hours for this exercise. This exercise should be done in conjunction with Exercise 8 'Using the assessment model', which will take a further hour. It is suggested that a half-day be allocated for the two exercises.

Materials

- Flipchart paper and marker pens
- Pens and paper
- HO 13a and HO 13b: Queenie Bird, or HO 14a and HO 14b: Walter Mumford

N.B. This exercise requires the trainer or someone who is not part of the learning group to take the role of the service user.

Trainer's guidelines

Step 1: allow 15 minutes
Introduce the exercise. Explain to the group that they are going to be involved in a collective assessment of a service user, role-played by yourself or someone

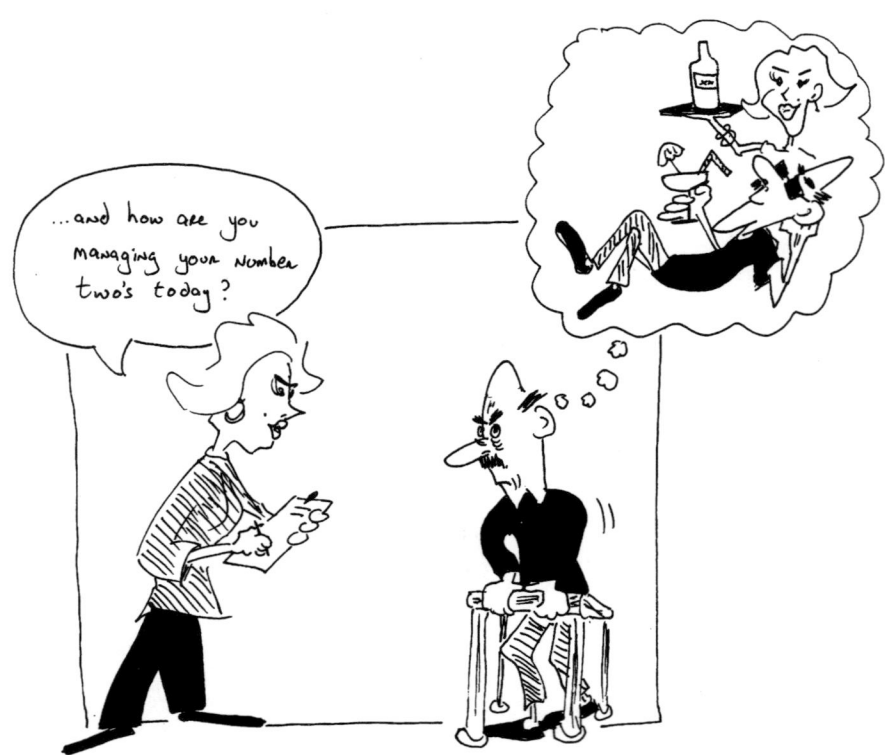

else who is not part of the learning group. Divide the participants into groups of three to four individuals. This exercise is ideally undertaken with four groups, each group having three to four members. Give out HO 13a or HO 14a. Allow the participants time to read the information and then briefly discuss in their groups what they think would be the typical response to this sort of referral. Emphasise that you are not looking for the ideal response, only the likely response.

Step 2: allow 10 minutes
Ask the groups what response would be likely in the circumstances. Explain that you have further information about the service user in the form of a second hand-out, which you then give out. It is on the basis of this further information that they will be interviewing the individual.

Step 3: allow 15 minutes
Participants prepare in their groups the questions they want to ask the service user in order to assess the individual's needs. Explain that you will go into role and begin by turning to Group 1 and allowing them between 5–10 minutes. During this time the other groups will act as observers. You will then move on to Group 2 and allow them between 5–10 minutes and so on until all of the groups have had a turn. At the end you will allow any further questions from any of the groups in order to ensure all questions have been asked. Obviously groups will not need to go over areas that have already been covered by previous groups, although they may feel there is perhaps a particular question that still needs to be asked. Reassure participants that, although it might sound a rather contrived exercise, it does actually work. I would suggest leaving each group to decide who will ask the questions. They may nominate one person, or they may all join in.

I first did this exercise on the basis of doing the role-plays with each group separately. This takes much longer, the other groups get restless waiting for their turn, and it can result in different information being obtained. And so I developed the idea of the collective interview, where everyone can listen at the same time to what is being said. This also ensures that everyone has heard the same information and is identifying the needs on a consistent basis.

Step 4: allow 30 minutes
Go into role and allow each group to ask their questions. Not all trainers will feel entirely comfortable with this method, and you might want to ask someone to play the role for you. The important point is to familiarise yourself with the case sheet details and then allow yourself to settle into the character, so that you can respond spontaneously to questions, and also volunteer comments and observations. It can make the exercise both more fun and more real if you not only provide information to the group, but also express your feelings in role about your situation and the questions you are being asked.

Step 5: allow 15 minutes
After the interview has concluded, return to your training role and ask the participants in their groups to identify the service user's needs.

Step 6: allow 35 minutes

Ask the groups in turn to identify one of the service user's needs. Write each need on the flipchart. Ask the participants to think about how the need is being written. Are they slipping into a service led approach, e.g. they need home care? There are always difficulties around areas where further investigation is needed. The health needs fall into this category, and so participants will often say the service user needs to see the doctor or the occupational therapist. It is important to distinguish between what is a service user need and what is required to meet the need effectively. So the service user's need may be 'to move around the house safely and independently' but, in order to meet that need, it may be necessary for the occupational therapist to make an assessment. This may seem a little pedantic to some participants, but it is important in ensuring a service user focus in the assessment process.

The exact wording of the needs may have to be reviewed. Is the language appropriate for the service user? Will they understand it? Might they be offended or upset by the way they see their needs described? How, for instance, is the issue of incontinence written? Reassure participants that these are not always easy questions to answer.

Keep going round the groups until all the needs have been identified. Number each need as you write it up.

This completes the first part of the two part exercise.

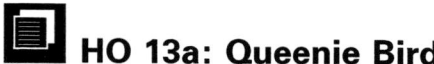 **HO 13a: Queenie Bird**

Preliminary information

Background and family circumstances (given by Gloria, the daughter-in law)

Mrs Queenie Bird is an 83-year-old woman who has lived in Worthing, Sussex since 1983, after moving from London with Bernard, her husband, who worked as a solicitor. Bernard died of an aortic aneurism in 1995. Queenie brought up four children, three boys and a daughter. She never worked outside the home.

Kathy, the daughter, aged 50, lives abroad with her husband and three children in Canada. Nigel, the eldest son, aged 60, has a heart problem. He used to be a keen sportsman, and is increasingly depressed over his failing health. He lives in Glasgow with his second wife, Maria, who is Columbian. They have no children. Colin, aged 57, works as a head teacher, and is off work suffering from stress. He is hoping to get early retirement. His two grown-up children are still living at home with him in London. His wife Deirdre died two years ago. Simon, aged 53, manages his own manufacturing business and lives in Portsmouth. He is very busy and has financial problems. His wife, Gloria works as a police officer and they have two daughters, who are both at university.

Domestic circumstances and social contact

Queenie owns her own three bedroom house and has a private pension from her late husband. She looks forward to family visits, but the children don't come as often as she would like, and when they do come they are often tired and preoccupied with their own problems. All her children ring her each week.

Queenie has few friends where she now lives, except for Penny, who has cleaned for her for 15 years and comes in twice a week. Penny is aged 75. Queenie has kept in touch with her old friends in London, most of whom are now very frail. Queenie travelled up to London to see them quite regularly until ten years ago. The visits then became less and less frequent, and now she relies on the phone. She likes to go out walking, and this, together with reading the newspaper, are her main interests.

Areas of concern

Queenie has enjoyed good health most of her life, although she has developed some weakness of the bladder at night, but she feels she is managing the problem. She is prone to digestive problems and does not always bother to get herself a meal. She often eats in a local café, but she is finding that is becoming more expensive. Queenie has become more anxious recently and the doctor has prescribed her anti-depressants.

Gloria, her daughter-in-law, has rung social services, and said that she is worried that Queenie is becoming more isolated and lonely, and might benefit from attending a day centre. Gloria is also concerned about her mother-in-law's irregular eating habits, and has requested meals on wheels.

HO 13b: Follow-up information

Queenie agreed to visit the day centre once and hated it. She said it was too noisy. She also agreed to meals on wheels, but then did not answer the door when they called. Queenie said that she didn't know when they were coming, and so was either out or still asleep. She said she didn't want to continue with them.

Gloria has called to say that Queenie has had a fall in the street and injured her mouth and right hand. Penny has gone away on holiday, and Queenie does not know when she is returning. Gloria is concerned that her mother-in-law is not eating properly and living on toast. She is also worried that the injury to Queenie's arm has prevented her from leaving the house since the fall.

When you visit Queenie at home it is a very cold day and the central heating is not switched on. Queenie is coughing. You notice a strong smell of urine coming from her bedroom and find urine all over the toilet floor. The bathroom and kitchen are not particularly clean and stale cat food has been left in a saucer.

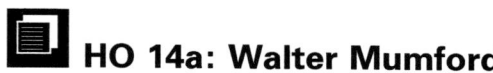 **HO 14a: Walter Mumford**

Preliminary information (provided by Gordon Priest, a neighbour and former friend)

Background information

Walter Mumford is a 55-year-old white man. He lives alone in a ground floor flat that he owns in Manchester. He was the only son from a mining family from the north-east. He has never married, and has no family with whom he is in contact. He has had a variety of jobs, mostly semi-skilled. He worked as a traffic warden for ten years until he was dismissed five years ago after getting into a fight with a member of the public while on duty. He has not worked since then.

Domestic circumstances and social contact

He spends a lot of time on his own at home. He has a neighbour, Gordon Priest who lives in the first floor flat in the same house, with whom he used to be good friends. Relations have become increasingly strained since Walter lost his job.

Areas of concern

Gordon is worried about Walter and phoned social services, saying that he thinks Walter needs help because he is not himself. Gordon says that whenever he knocks on Walter's door he just gets a 'load of abuse'. He doesn't think Walter is looking after himself or the flat properly. Gordon says that he knows Walter has had his gas and electricity cut off. When you ring, Walter tells you 'to mind you own business'.

HO 14b: Follow-up information

Gordon rings you to say that Walter was attacked by intruders, who broke into his flat. Walter was badly beaten up and has been left with a broken right arm and two broken ribs (Walter is right-handed). After two days Walter was discharged from hospital, saying to staff that he would be able to manage at home.

Gordon has rung the office to say that after visiting Walter in his home, he believes Walter needs help. Their friendship has been revived after Gordon called the police and the ambulance when Walter was attacked.

Gordon describes Walter as living 'in squalor'. He believes Walter has 'neglected himself and is depressed'. Gordon says he has tried to help but he feels Walter needs more professional support. Gordon says he doesn't mind doing a bit of shopping for Walter, but he works away and so isn't always around to help. Walter has agreed to see you.

When you arrive, the flat is cold, and despite evidence of Gordon's attempts to clear up, there is still a lot of rubbish lying around. The kitchen and bathroom do not appear to have been cleaned for a long time. The sink, bath and toilet are heavily stained and the pattern on both vinyl floors is no longer distinguishable. Carpets are encrusted with trodden in food.

Section C: We know where we're going

The problem with objectives

Writing objectives can be a confusing business and, even worse from the practitioner's standpoint, it can also seem a singular waste of time. Many will say that their main concern is to get the service in as quickly as possible, and all the form-filling seems to just complicate the process and make for unnecessary delay. Indeed the service users themselves may echo this frustration.

So perhaps it is worth acknowledging that the paperwork and the systems of assessment can sometimes involve a degree of duplication. It is a problem that single, shared or unified assessment should, when fully implemented, go some way to address.

The issue of distinguishing needs, objectives and services in the assessment process is distinct from the issue of overly cumbersome forms. It is about ensuring that we are clear about the purpose of our intervention with a service user, and that the most appropriate and effective response has been identified. Explicit objective setting ultimately benefits service users, in that their needs are more precisely understood, and it also benefits service providers, in that they are clearer about what is expected of them. It also benefits agencies responsible for the provision of those services to service users, in that the parties agree realistic, measurable, relevant yardsticks by which the effectiveness of the services in meeting needs can be evaluated.

While objective setting will not magically increase levels of provision, or introduce services that are not currently available, it will help in giving a clearer account of how service users are being supported. This then provides the evidence for making a more effective argument as to how that support could be improved.

It is acknowledged that assessment and care planning cover a much broader area than is being attempted in this context. The focus here is simply on how assessments are recorded and in particular the issue of writing objectives. This material assumes that the broad principles of good practice in assessment are already understood.

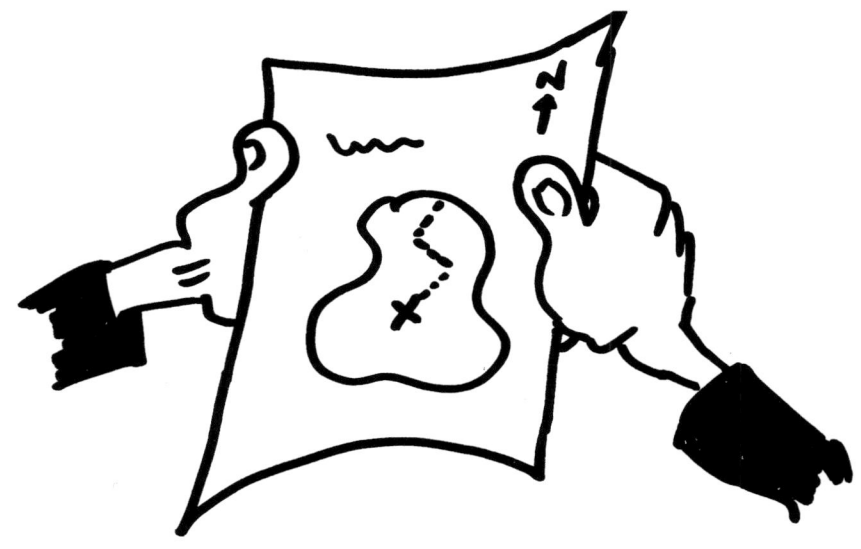

The models of assessment

It will be helpful to look at two models of objective setting and compare their relative value.

The evaluation model

Need 1. Identify need. *e.g. Continued contact with wife while she is in hospital.*	→	**Service** 2. Identify who can meet the need. *e.g. Daughter and volunteer provide transport.*	→	**Outcome/objective** 3. Identify how you will know if the need has been met. *e.g. Visited wife twice a week.*

In this model the setting of the outcome or objective has become a means of evaluating the effectiveness of the service intervention. Once the need has been identified, the focus moves on to what services should be used, without exploring what has to be done in order to meet the need. The objective is only stated after the service provision has been decided.

The assessment model

Need 1. Identify need. *e.g. Continued contact with wife while she is in hospital.*	→	**Outcome/objective** 2. What has to be done to meet the need? *e.g. To visit wife in hospital twice a week.*	→	**Service** 3. Who can meet the need? *e.g. Daughter and volunteer each takes Mr A to hospital once a week.*

In this model the setting of the objective is not an afterthought to the process, it is central to the process and to the way in which the assessment is conducted. There is a logical progression from identifying need, to deciding what has to be done to meet the need, and only then considering who or what service might be most appropriate to meet that need.

The assessment model provides greater flexibility in exploring the different ways in which a need might be met. In the example used of the gentleman wanting to maintain contact with his wife while in hospital, the objectives could have also included telephone calls on the days he did not visit. He may or may not have needed assistance with this particular objective, but it would have been useful to include, and it also underlines the service user as an active participant in the process, not just a recipient of help from others.

Exercise 8: Using the assessment model

(This exercise is a continuation from 'Whose need is it anyway?')

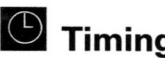 **Objective**

To define outcome/objectives from identified needs.

 Timing

Allow 1 hour for this exercise

 Materials needed

- Overhead projector
- OHT 2: Defining objectives
- OHT 3: Writing objectives
- OHT 4: Effective objectives need to be SMART
- OHT 5: Common problems: Rewriting needs
- OHT 6: Common problems: Service objectives
- OHT 7: Common problems: Action planning
- Flipchart, and marker pens
- Pens and paper
- HO 15: Defining objectives
- HO 16: Common problems

 Trainer's guidelines

Step 1: allow 20 minutes
Present OHT 2: Defining objectives
OHT 3: Writing objectives
OHT 4: Effective objectives need to be SMART
OHT 5: Common problems: Rewriting needs
OHT 6: Common problems: Service objectives
OHT 7: Common problems: Action planning

Step 2: allow 15 minutes
Ask participants working in the same groups they were in for 'Whose need is it anyway?' to select four of the needs identified in the review discussion at the end of the last exercise. Ask them to now write the objectives from those needs. It doesn't matter which needs each group select, or if they select the same or different needs. Explain that, for practical purposes, it is assumed that they have already discussed and agreed the objectives with the service user concerned. Ask them to write the objectives, matching the number of the objective to the number given to the need, to ensure everyone knows to which need the different objectives refer.

Step 3: allow 25 minutes
Bring the groups back together. Ask each group in turn to read out which need they addressed, and then read out the objective from the need. If any of the

other groups have also covered that particular need you can ask them for their version. Write each of these versions on the flipchart and then evaluate how effectively they each work as an objective. Is it written in terms of what the service user will do? Is it written in language the service user will understand? Is it sufficiently precise in terms of SMART principles? It may be necessary to rewrite the objective in discussion with the groups. Continue working in turn through the objectives written by each group until all have been covered and satisfactorily stated.

OHT 2: Defining objectives

All objectives should be discussed and agreed with the service user or, where the service user cannot meaningfully be involved, with the service user's representative.

Objectives can be:

● **Developmental**

Enabling people to move forward, improving quality of life, learning or regaining skills, achieving new goals, e.g. improving ability to get about.

● **Maintenance**

Supporting people to continue with existing quality of life. Retaining current level of functioning, e.g. being clean and comfortable.

● **Preventative**

Ensuring people's situation does not deteriorate. Reducing risks, protecting people from the potentially damaging consequences of the need not being met, e.g. taking prescribed medication.

OHT 3: Writing objectives

- **Be positive**

  Objectives should always be positively stated. Write what someone *will* be doing rather than what they *will not* be doing. e.g. H will join in with one social activity each week, *rather than* H will not spend all his time in his room.

- **Put the service user first**

  Remember it is always the service user who achieves the objective. This is helped by starting the sentence with the service user, even when assistance may be required. e.g. H will eat a daily lunch time meal, prepared by one other.

- **Be specific**

  State clearly what it is the service user will be doing, in terms of observable behaviour. Think about which verb best describes the service user's action. e.g. H *will* wash (or *dress*, or *walk* to the park, or *collect* newspaper) daily.

- **State the conditions**

  What conditions are required for achieving the objective? Can the service user act independently or do they need support? e.g. H will use the toilet:

  o independently

  o using stated equipment

  o under supervision

  o with verbal prompts

  o with assistance from one other

  o in the company of another person

OHT 4: Effective objectives need to be:

<u>S</u>pecific

Clear and precise as to what is to be done.

<u>M</u>easurable

It is possible to say to what extent the objective has been achieved.

<u>A</u>greed

With the user and with other parties involved.

<u>R</u>ealistic

Achievable within the resources available.

<u>T</u>ime related

Specifies by when and how often the objective should be achieved.

OHT 5: Common problems: rewriting needs

This is where workers simply try and find a different form of words to the stated need.

Example 1

Need

To be able to move around their home safely and independently.

Objective as rewritten need

To maintain their mobility inside their home.

Objective (which states how needs will be met)

To walk around their house, using their zimmer frame and to go up and down stairs using a stair-lift.

Example 2

Need

To be safe and secure in own home.

Objective as rewritten need

To maintain security in the home.

Objective (which states how needs will be met)

To allow others secure access to the home with the use of a key-safe.

Example 3

Need

To develop social contacts in the local community.

Objective as rewritten need

To have opportunities to meet people in local community.

Objective (which states how needs will be met)

To go to bingo in the company of another each week.

OHT 6: Common problems: service objectives

This is where the objectives are stated more in terms of what the service provider will be doing rather than the service user. This problem is more likely when the need is expressed in terms of 'help to' or 'assistance with'.

Example 1

Need

Help to wash and dress.

Service objective

To help client with personal care.

User objective (which states how needs will be met)

To shower daily and dress with the help of one other, with the opportunity to choose own clothes.

Example 2

Need

Assistance with shopping.

Service objective

To ensure client has adequate supplies of food and groceries.

User objective (which states how needs will be met)

To make a weekly shopping list of food and groceries which will be purchased by one other, or, to visit the local shops weekly accompanied by another.

Example 3

Need

Assistance with medication.

Service objective

To help client take medication as prescribed.

User objective (which states how needs will be met)

To use blister pack medication with the prompting of one other.

OHT 7: Common problems: action planning

This is where the objectives have become a little more than an action plan for the worker.

Example 1

Need

To have a regular and balanced diet.

Objective as action plan

Arrange Meals on Wheels.

Objective (which states how needs will be met)

To eat daily, breakfast prepared by themself, lunch time meal and sandwiches at tea time prepared by another.

Example 2

Need

To come to terms with loss of husband.

Objective as action plan

Refer to counselling.

Objective (which states how needs will be met)

To have the opportunity to talk about feelings following death of husband.

Example 3

Need

To get in and out of the bath.

Objective as action plan

Refer to occupational therapist.

Objective (which states how needs will be met)

To bath every other day using a hoist assisted by two others.

HO 15: Defining objectives

All objectives should be discussed and agreed with the service user, or where the service user cannot meaningfully be involved, with the service user's representative.

Objectives can be:

- **Developmental**
  Enabling people to move forward, improving quality of life, learning or regaining skills, achieving new goals. e.g. improving ability to get about.
- **Maintenance**
  Supporting people to continue with existing quality of life. Retaining current level of functioning. e.g. being clean and comfortable.
- **Preventative**
  Ensuring people's situations do not deteriorate. Reducing risks, protecting people from the potentially damaging consequences of the need not being met, e.g. taking prescribed medication.

Effective objectives need to be:

- **Specific**
  Clear and precise as to what is to be done.
- **Measurable**
  It is possible to say to what extent the objective has been achieved.
- **Agreed**
  With the user and with other parties involved.
- **Realistic**
  Achievable within the resources available.
- **Time related**
  Specifies by when and how often the objective should be achieved.

Writing objectives:

- **Be positive**
  Objectives should always be positively stated. Write what someone *will* be doing rather than what they *will* not be doing, e.g. H will join in with one social activity each week, *rather than*, H will not spend all his time in his room.
- **Put the service user first**
  Remember it is always the service user who achieves the objective. This is helped by starting the sentence with the service user, even when assistance may be required, e.g. H will eat a daily lunch time meal prepared by one other.
- **Be specific**
  State clearly what it is the service user will be doing, in terms of observable behaviour. Think about which verb best describes the service user's action, e.g. H will wash (or dress, or walk to the park, or collect newspaper) daily.
- **State the conditions**
  What conditions are required for achieving the objective? Can the service user act independently or do they need support?

e.g. H will use the toilet:
  ○ independently
  ○ using stated equipment
  ○ under supervision
  ○ with verbal prompts
  ○ with assistance from one other
  ○ in the company of another person

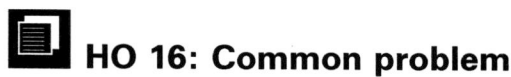 **HO 16: Common problems**

Common problems: rewriting needs

This is where workers simply try and find a different form of words to the stated need.

Example 1

Need

To be able to move around their home safely and independently.

Objective as rewritten need

To maintain their mobility inside their home.

Objective (which states how needs will be met)

To walk around their house using their zimmer frame, and to go up and down stairs using a stair-lift.

Example 2

Need

To be safe and secure in own home.

Objective as rewritten need

To maintain security in the home.

Objective (which states how needs will be met)

To allow others secure access to the home with the use of a key-safe.

Example 3

Need

To develop social contacts in the local community.

Objective as rewritten need

To have opportunities to meet people in local community.

Objective (which states how needs will be met)

To go to bingo in the company of another each week.

Common problems – service objectives

This is where the objectives are stated more in terms of what the service provider will be doing rather than the service user. This problem is more likely when the need is expressed in terms of 'help to' or 'assistance with'.

Example 1

Need

Help to wash and dress.

Service objective

To help client with personal care.

User objective (which states how the need will be met)

To shower daily and dress with the help of one other, with the opportunity to choose own clothes.

Example 2

Need

Assistance with shopping.

Service objective

To ensure client has adequate supplies of food and groceries.

User objective (which states how the need will be met)

To make a weekly shopping list of food and groceries which will be purchased by one other.
To visit the local shops weekly accompanied by another.

Example 3

Need

Assistance with medication.

Service objective

To help client take medication as prescribed.

User objective (which states how the need will be met)

To use blister pack medication with the prompting of one other.

Common problems – action planning

This is where the objectives have become a little more than an action plan for the worker.

Example 1

Need

To have a regular and balanced diet.

Objective as action plan

Arrange Meals on Wheels.

Objective (which states how the need will be met)

To eat daily, breakfast prepared by himself, lunch time meal and sandwiches at tea time prepared by another.

Example 2

Need

To come to terms with loss of husband.

Objective as action plan

Refer to counselling.

Objective (which states how the need will be met)

To have the opportunity to talk about feelings following death of husband.

Example 3

Need

To get in and out of the bath.

Objective as action plan

Refer to occupational therapist.

Objective (which states how the need will be met)

To bath every other day using a hoist assisted by two others.

Chapter 3: The Bus Principle

This chapter refers to the proverbial bus, under which practitioners are light-heartedly reminded they may one day fall, and asked how adequate their records would be, in that event, for anyone else to pick up and work with. This has the effect of underlining to practitioners that they are essentially writing to communicate to someone else, rather than simply providing a record of their own work. They are sharing the information they have been given by the service user and others, and organising that information into a coherent account that will adequately tell the story to anyone else who subsequently works with that service user. Single, shared or unified assessments will emphasise even more the importance of providing sufficient information about a service user in the assessment. The care co-ordinator's responsibility in single, shared or unified assessments is to ensure that information is only given once, and the service user does not have to repeat their story to every new professional or practitioner they encounter.

The chapter has two sections, 'It's a long story' and 'It's obvious isn't it?'

Section A: It's a long story

One of the greatest difficulties practitioners describe is how to judge what level of detail they should include in a written account. Certainly the wish to be more concise is probably top of most participants' lists of learning expectations, when they come on recording skills training. In the same way, a major criticism of case recording is that important information is often buried in irrelevant detail.

Practitioners have a great deal of information from which to select, much of which may be held in their heads as supporting material. This may make it very difficult for them to recognise what they themselves know at an almost intuitive level. It may then require a very considerable and conscious effort to provide sufficient detail, to ensure that the story can be understood by the reader in the

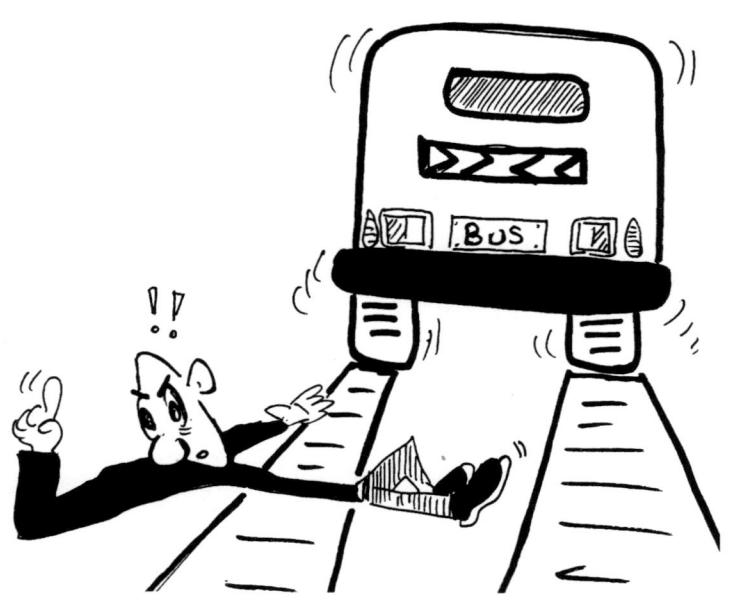

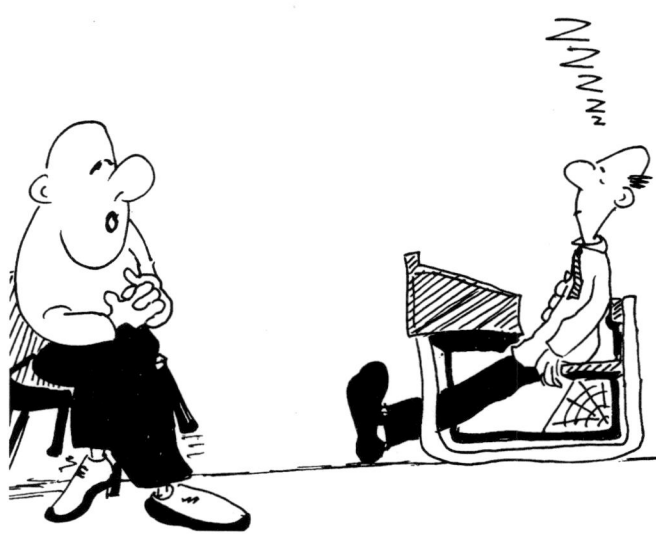

way that the writer understands it. Many of us have the problem of not necessarily making all our implied assumptions explicit when we try to describe something to someone else. The familiar experience of trying to give someone directions serves as an example. We struggle to think in terms of the perspective of our readers or listeners, who do not, like us, have the background information, who will not know what we mean unless we tell them. So we try to decide how much detail to include, aware that too much information can be as much of an obstacle to understanding as too little.

The material is designed to allow participants to compare two accounts of the same service user. The 'War and Peace' version includes a lot of unnecessary detail which obscures the important issues. The 'short and sweet' version provides only the barest information and would leave the service user having to repeat their story to each new worker they encounter. A 'does the job' version is provided as a guide to what information should be included. It is not meant to be prescriptive, and should serve as a guide or comparison to the versions produced by the participants.

Exercise 9: The three versions

 Objective

To evaluate what information should be included in order to provide an adequate and relevant account of a service user and their situation.

 Timing

Allow 1 ½ hours for this exercise

 Materials

- HO 18a, HO 18b and HO 18c: Farah Ali Ahmet
- or HO 19a, HO 19b and HO 19c: Lionel Jenkins
- Pens and paper
- Flipchart paper and marker pens
- Overhead projector
- OHT 8, 9

ⓘ Trainer's guidelines

Step 1: allow 15 minutes
Show OHT 8 and OHT 9
   Acknowledge the difficulties that many workers experience in trying to decide how much information is relevant to include in a written account of a service user. Explain that OHT 8 identifies the main questions to address in deciding whether an account is sufficient. OHT 9 illustrates the way in which too much and too little information can both create problems.
   Give out HOs.

Step 2: allow 5 minutes
Introduce the exercise and split the participants into groups of three or four members. Give out the case sheets of the 'War and Peace' version and the 'short and sweet' version of the character selected. Ask the participants to discuss what information would need to be included in the 'does the job' version. Explain that you want them to write the 'does the job' version in note form on flipchart paper.

Step 3: allow 45 minutes
Allow participants to write the 'does the job' version.

Step 4: allow 25 minutes
Put each piece of flipchart paper on the wall and ask each group to read through what they have written and to explain why they decided to include the information they did. As they do this you may want to clarify why certain details were included, or not. After all the groups have read out and explained their accounts, you may then like to compare them with the suggested 'does the job' version and ask participants to comment.

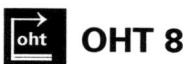 **OHT 8**

Problems identified with case recording

- Relevant information buried in irrelevant detail

How do you decide what information should be included?

- Has the reader sufficient information to understand the service user's needs?

- Can the reader hear the service user's account of what has happened to them and why?

- Will the service user have to tell their story again to each new practitioner they see?

- Is all the information relevant to understanding the service user and their situation?

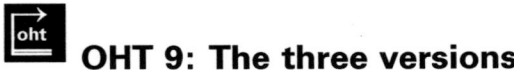 **OHT 9: The three versions**

The 'War and Peace' version

Provides too much information, in that many details do not add to any more significant understanding of the service user, or the experiences, which may have contributed to their present situation.

The 'short and sweet' version

Provides an essential summary of the service user's situation, but does not include enough information to understand how and why the person came to be in their present situation.

With only the barest details, the service user would have to repeat their story to each new worker they encountered.

The 'does the job' version

Provides sufficient information to enable other practitioners to understand the service user, and how and why they came to be in their present situation, without the service having to repeat the same details to each new practitioner.

HO 17: The bus principle

Problems identified with case recording:

● Relevant information buried in irrelevant detail

How do you decide what information should be included?

● Has the reader sufficient information to understand the service user's needs?
● Can the reader hear the service user's account of what has happened to them and why?
● Will the service user have to tell their story again to each new practitioner they see?
● Is all the information relevant to understanding the service user and their situation?

The three versions

The 'War and Peace' version

Provides too much information, in that many details do not add to any more significant understanding of the service user, or the experiences, which may have contributed to their present situation.

The 'short and sweet' version

Provides an essential summary of the service user's situation, but does not include enough information to understand how and why the person came to be in their present situation.

With only the barest details, the service user would have to repeat their story to each new worker they encountered.

The 'does the job' version

Provides sufficient information to enable other practitioners to understand the service user, and how and why they came to be in their present situation, without the service having to repeat the same details to each new practitioner.

HO 18a: Farah Ali Ahmed: The 'War and Peace' version

Farah Ali Ahmed is 34-years-old. He was born in Somalia in 1970 and grew up during a period of great turmoil in his country's history. His family, who are Muslim, were opposed to Siad Barre, who took control of the country through a military coup in 1969. Farah and various male relatives, including his father, who worked as a teacher, and his three brothers, joined the Somali National Movement, which rose up in 1988 against Siad Barre. The SNM was brutally suppressed, and many of Farah's family were killed, including his father and two of his brothers. His other brother disappeared.

Farah himself was eventually arrested in 1989, and tortured over a six-month period, during which he received regular beatings. He says they did other things that he is still unable to talk about. In 1990 he escaped from prison and then went into hiding. It was then that he learned that his mother had also died in the fighting. He had two sisters but they had disappeared. It was thought they had been abducted by government troops. Farah says elder members of his clan paid for him to travel to Kenya and then fly out from Kenya on forged papers. He sought asylum in Britain in January 1991.

He says that he found it very difficult at first, because he did not know anyone and his English was not very good. He was in a poor state of health, and was hospitalised with pneumonia at one point. He lived in one room in London, and said that for the first year he hardly spoke to anyone. He then made friends with some fellow Somalis who had also fled to Britain.

It took three years for his asylum application to be processed. There were various administrative delays, which Farah didn't understand, which meant that he was unable to work legally during that period, and would have had to depend on benefit, had it not been for a contact who told him about places where people would not ask too many questions. He got a job as a cleaner in a hotel. This meant he could send some money home to his sisters, with whom he had established contact again.

After his asylum application had been accepted, he said he was able to start rebuilding his life properly. He said he felt secure for the first time in his life. His English had improved sufficiently and he got a job as a postman. He said that he enjoyed the work until he was put under pressure by other Somalis to be involved in a scam in which credit cards were being stolen as they were sent through the post. He said he didn't want to do this, but he felt he didn't have much choice. He was told by gang members that if he didn't join in, they would denounce him to the Home Office and he would be deported. In 1995 the ringleaders of the scam were caught by the police, and Farah was given the opportunity of immunity from prosecution if he testified against them. As the only alternative was prosecution and deportation he agreed. He was given 'witness protection' in the period leading up to the trial. He says he found this very difficult, as he couldn't leave where he was staying and he felt very frightened all the time. After the trial, the police advised him to move from London and take on a new identity, to escape a revenge attack. He was put in contact with a community worker with the Somali community in Liverpool who arranged discreet accommodation for him, living with a local Somali family.

Farah said he knew that the people he testified against had very powerful friends, and so he was constantly looking over his shoulder. He said he began to think that he would never feel safe anywhere. He said the family he was living with were very kind and treated him like a son. Eventually he got a job in a bottling plant. In 1999 he married the eldest daughter of the family with whom he was staying.

Farah and his wife moved out into their own flat in 2000. They had a son in 2001 and a daughter in 2003. Farah said his wife contracted TB after the birth of the second baby, and this made things very difficult. At the same time Farah was made redundant. He says he tried hard to find other work, but all he was offered was very low paid cleaning jobs. Within a few months they were forced to move back in with his wife's parents. Farah said that his wife started blaming him for their problems. He says they were always arguing and he sometimes lost his temper, and on occasions he did hit her. He said that he did not feel it was right for her to criticise him in front of her parents. He felt humiliated. He said that her parents would take her side in the arguments, and eventually he had enough and walked out. He says that his wife has made it impossible for him to see his children, and he does not understand why she is allowed to do this. He says she has started divorce proceedings.

After he left his wife, he moved in with an Algerian friend. One evening two months ago, while returning from the mosque, they were set upon by a group of white and black youths who attacked them with knives, shouting anti-Muslim abuse. There had recently been arrests in the area of young Muslims on suspicion of terrorist activity. Farah says that he has experienced some hostility ever since he came to Britain, including some low level violence, but it was 'not that bad'. He did feel that this time it was different. They seemed more extreme. His friend sustained fairly superficial injuries, but Farah, after he fell to the ground, was kicked repeatedly in the head as well as receiving several stab wounds to the chest. After emergency surgery Farah survived, although he has sustained serious visual impairment in both eyes. He is still in hospital. His friend says he is unable to have him return with him. Farah's wife has said he is nothing to do with her any more.

Farah appears anxious and depressed. He says he does not want to live anymore, that he will not be able to look after himself. He says he does not want people's pity. He feels that even when he was in Somalia he did not face such a desperate situation as he does now. Nursing staff have said that Farah has shown no interest in a programme of rehabilitation. They say he spends most of his time asleep or lying on his bed doing nothing.

According to the medical reports Farah has made a good recovery from the wounds to his chest. One of his lungs was punctured, but that has now healed and, while he may take some time to regain full fitness, he is ready for discharge. The medical staff are less certain about the prognosis in relation to the damage to his sight. This resulted from injury to the brain and the optic nerve rather than the eyes. There is the possibility that in time he may recover some partial vision, but it is too early to say with any degree of confidence.

Having discussed his situation with him it seems that Farah is overwhelmed by what has happened to him and is unable to cope. He says that he has no future, although when the question of discharge from hospital is raised, he simply says 'Do with me what you will. I do not care anymore. There is nothing left.'

I believe Farah will require substantial support on leaving hospital in order to come to terms with and cope with his disability. I feel that his sense of hopelessness is understandable in terms of what has happened to him during his life. He has had to contend with many extreme circumstances that would be beyond the emotional resources of many. However, he seems to have got to a point where he may require, in addition to help with his sensory disability, professional support with his feelings of despair.

I would therefore recommend that, in order to plan an effective discharge from hospital, support from both the mental health team and sensory impairment team be put in place, along with arranging suitable accommodation. It may be worth considering a temporary residential placement which could address all these needs together and provide an effective programme of rehabilitation. I have suggested this to Farah and he says that he 'is in our hands' and will do whatever we think is best.

HO 18b: Farah Ali Ahmed: The 'short and sweet' version

Current situation

Farah Ali Ahmed, aged 34, came to Britain from Somalia in 1991. He has been in hospital for two months, after being attacked and receiving stab wounds to the chest and blows to the head. He has severe visual impairment in both eyes.

He is separated from his wife and two children, and was previously living with a friend. His friend is unable to have him return with him.

While Farah is ready for discharge, he shows little interest in any programmes of rehabilitation. He appears very low in mood and does not seem to care what happens to him.

Background information

Before coming to Britain, Farah lost most of his family in Somalia, and was himself imprisoned and tortured. After his asylum application was accepted in 1994, Farah worked in London. He later moved to Liverpool, where he married and had two children. The relationship broke down and divorce proceedings are pending.

Immediate needs

Medical staff have suggested that he needs a mental health assessment, and from my own observations I believe that Farah will be at risk without mental health support.

In addition he will require assessment by the sensory impairment team and a rehabilitation programme. Accommodation will need to be arranged before he can be discharged.

In my opinion a temporary residential placement should be considered.

▣ HO 18c: Farah Ali Ahmed: The 'does the job' version

Current situation

Farah Ali Ahmed is aged 34 and came to Britain from Somalia in 1991. He has been in hospital for two months after being attacked by an anti-Muslim gang. He received stab wounds to the chest and blows to the head, which resulted in a punctured lung and severe visual impairment in both eyes.

He is separated from his wife and two children, aged three years and twelve months. Farah was previously living with a friend. His friend is unable to have him return with him.

While Farah is ready for discharge, he shows little interest in any programmes of rehabilitation. He appears very low in mood and does not seem to care what happens to him, saying, 'Do with me what you will. I do not care anymore. There is nothing left.'

Background information

Before coming to Britain, Farah's family, who are Muslim, were involved in an uprising in 1988, during which he lost many members of his family, including his parents and two brothers. The remaining brother and two sisters disappeared. Farah was imprisoned and tortured for six months. He says he still cannot talk about everything that happened during this period. He escaped from prison and was helped by members of his clan to reach Britain, where he applied for asylum. His application took three years, during which time he earned extra money on top of his benefit, working illegally in order to send money to his sisters, with whom he was again in contact. His health suffered, and he was hospitalised with pneumonia.

After his asylum application was accepted in 1994, Farah worked with the Post Office, which he says he enjoyed until he was forced by other Somalis to be involved in a credit card scam. He was told by gang members that if he didn't join in, they would denounce him to the Home Office and he would be deported. In 1995 the ringleaders of the gang were arrested and Farah was offered immunity if he testified against them. As the only alternative was prosecution and deportation, he agreed. He was given 'witness protection' before the trial. He says he felt very frightened during this time. After the trial, the police advised him to leave London and assume a new identity. He moved to Liverpool and a community worker arranged for him to live with a local Somali family.

In 1999 he married the eldest daughter of the family with whom he was staying. They moved into a flat a year later. A son was born in 2001 and a daughter in 2003, after which his wife contracted TB and Farah was made redundant. They moved back in with his wife's family. He said he and his wife were always arguing, he felt humiliated and occasionally he hit her. Tensions built up to a point where he walked out. He says his wife has made it impossible for him to see his children, and she has started divorce proceedings.

Immediate needs

According to the medical reports Farah has made a good recovery. His punctured lung has healed and, while he may take some time to regain full fitness, he is ready for discharge. The medical staff are less certain about the prognosis in relation to the damage to his sight. This resulted from injury to the brain and the optic nerve. There is the possibility that in time he may recover some partial vision, but it is too early to say with any degree of confidence.

Farah says he does not want to live anymore, that he will not be able to look after himself. He says he does not want people's pity. He feels that even when he was in Somalia he did not face such a desperate situation as he does now. Nursing staff have said that Farah has shown no interest in a programme of rehabilitation. They say he spends most of his time asleep or lying on his bed doing nothing.

I believe Farah will require substantial support on leaving hospital in order to come to terms with and cope with his disability. I feel that his sense of hopelessness is understandable in terms of what has happened to him during his life. Medical staff have suggested that he needs a mental health assessment, and from my own observations I believe that Farah will be at risk without mental health intervention.

In addition he will require assessment by the sensory impairment team, and a rehabilitation programme. Accommodation will need to be arranged before he can be discharged.

In view of concerns around Farah's low mood, his disability, and the need for rehabilitation, together with the immediate lack of accommodation, all of which put Farah at risk, it may be an option to consider a temporary residential placement which could address these various needs together. This has been discussed in principle with Farah, and he has agreed.

⬛ HO 19a: Lionel Jenkins: The 'War and Peace' version

Lionel Jenkins is an 82-year-old man who was born in Swansea, South Wales in 1922. He was the eldest of eight children. He says his family were close knit. His father worked as a crane driver, but it was his mother who held the family together through the Depression. Lionel says she was a very strong character, and he was her favourite.

Lionel developed TB when he was seventeen, at the outbreak of World War II. He spent most of the war in hospital, convalescing. It was during this time that he met his future wife Pearl, who worked as a nurse. Lionel said his mother never liked Pearl and this made things very difficult. He said that he had not really come to terms with not being able to fight in the war, and this, together with all the problems between his mother and Pearl, had all got too much and he had what he described as a 'nervous collapse'. He was in hospital for six months. After he came out of hospital, he and Pearl got married and his mother accepted the situation. Lionel got a job in the local bank.

Lionel said that he and Pearl had both looked forward to starting a family, and so it was a great disappointment when they found they were unable to have children. They decided to adopt. Harold, aged four months, arrived in 1947 and Dorothy, aged six months arrived in 1949. Lionel says that there were problems with Harold right from the beginning. He was always in trouble, whereas Dorothy was always a 'sweet child'. As an adult, Harold could never settle to anything. He married, but his wife left him because of his gambling. Lionel said it was a drain on him and his wife because they were forever trying to get Harold out of trouble. Lionel says it was just as well that he did quite well with his dabbling in the stock market as that enabled them to help Harold.

Lionel believes it was the worry over Harold that caused his wife's early death in 1981. She was only sixty. Lionel says that he found it very difficult to cope at the time, and that it was Brenda who helped him pull through. Brenda had been a friend to both Pearl and Lionel, and had helped nurse Pearl through the last year when she was dying of breast cancer. Lionel said that he had grown very close to Brenda through that time, and so they decided to get married. He says his children were not very pleased, because Brenda was a lot younger and they thought she was a gold-digger. He married Brenda in 1983, 18 months after his wife died. He retired in the same year.

Lionel says that it was not long after he married Brenda that his mother died. He missed her a great deal and, despite the problems between them, he had always had a very strong relationship with her. Lionel says that it was after this that he began to have problems eating in front of people. He says that he finds it difficult to swallow and he doesn't like having to eat in front of anyone. He didn't mind eating in front of Brenda, but not anyone else, including his children. Brenda accepted this, although Lionel acknowledges that this did make things difficult at times. Whenever they had visitors, he would take his meal in another room. Similarly it limited the people they could visit, as well as putting restrictions on the sort of holidays they could have. Lionel says that he realised this put a heavy burden on Brenda. Lionel says that she wanted him to get help, but he didn't want to see anyone about it. She stayed for ten years, but in the end she got fed up, and she left him in 1993 and went to live with her sister.

After Brenda left, Lionel lived on his own for about a year, but found it increasingly difficult to cope. In the end, his daughter, Dorothy, who has remained single, persuaded him to move nearer to where she was living in Bristol. Lionel said he found it very difficult moving from the house that he had lived in ever since he had married Pearl. He had never lived anywhere but in the Swansea area, except when he was convalescing during the war. He didn't have a large number of friends, because as he put it, 'he had never been a very sociable sort of person', but he did find it a 'terrible upheaval' although he accepted he was finding it difficult to manage on his own.

Dorothy found a small ground floor flat that was just round the corner from where she lived. Lionel says that Dorothy thought this was ideal, as he could still be independent, but she could keep an eye on him and make sure he had what he wanted. Dorothy would bring round meals for him and keep the place tidy. He was grateful to her, especially when he developed his heart condition. He said that he had had problems with his heart for a long time, but in the last few years it had become worse. His doctor told him he was suffering from a congestive heart. He is on medication, but Lionel says that he knows there isn't an awful lot they can do in the long run. He knows that he is too old for a heart transplant and so he just has to be 'grateful for whatever time he has left'.

Lionel says he 'doesn't know what he would have done without Dorothy'. Lionel says that she has been helping him to wash and dress and taking him out in the car. He still has the old problem of not being able to eat in front of anyone, and so they have had to take account of that. Lionel admits that he now has to wash his hands before he eats or drinks anything, including taking his medication, none of which he can do with anyone looking. He also requires Dorothy to wear a mask when she is preparing his food. He says he is not able to eat anything unless it has been prepared with these precautions.

Four weeks ago Dorothy was diagnosed with cancer of the liver. Lionel says that he had noticed that she had not been looking well, and that he had been worried about her. He says that she is trying to be positive, and she told him that the doctor said that they could try a new treatment, but Lionel says he knows that liver cancer is always fatal. He says it is just a question of how long. He says he can't bring himself to say that to Dorothy, because she is still trying to hold on to the idea that she will get better. However, he knows that she will no longer be able to look after him, and he knows he can't look after himself. He recognises that he is becoming weaker and weaker, with even very small exertions like going to the toilet, leaving him exhausted. He says he dreads being on his own after she has gone. Harold has said he can come and live with him, but Lionel said that he thinks his son is just interested in the little bit of money that Lionel has left. He has never trusted Harold and although he is his son, Lionel never wants to put himself in the position of being dependent on him.

Lionel says he has thought long and hard about it and has decided that the time has come to move into residential care. He says he would not like to continue living in the flat on his own after Dorothy has gone and he feels it would help her to know that he was alright. He says he would like to be able to keep some of his own things, like his bed and his chair and he would like to move back to Swansea so that he can 'end his days in his home town'.

He says that he needs help as soon as possible, as he doesn't want Dorothy worrying about him, and so he would like someone to come to the flat while he is waiting to find a place in a residential home in Swansea. He says he is particular about where he goes in Swansea, as he knows that there are some very 'rough' parts to the city. Lionel says that he owns his own flat, which he thinks is worth about £130,000, and that he still has about another £20,000 in savings and investments, despite having lost a considerable amount in recent years with all the problems in the stock market. He receives a pension from the bank on top of his state pension. He has also been claiming attendance allowance. Lionel says he wants help finding a home in Swansea. He knows that he will have to make a substantial contribution to the cost, but he says he doesn't mind as there is only Harold to leave anything to.

Lionel is concerned as to how far people will understand his particular needs around eating and drinking. He says it would be important for them to respect his problems and that he really could not eat anything unless it had been prepared according to his requirements. When this was pointed out as a potential area of difficulty, especially in a communal residential setting, Lionel said that he would have to insist his conditions were met. I suggested that it might be helpful if Lionel spoke to a psychologist who might be able to help him. Lionel was reluctant to pursue this.

In view of his daughter's situation, Lionel is now at risk without immediate assistance in both the areas of food preparation and personal care. Lionel will need support while still living in his flat in Bristol. Home Care would seem the most appropriate option, although staff would need to be made aware of Lionel's particular requirements around food preparation and eating and drinking. In the meantime it will be necessary to investigate residential care options in Swansea. Similar consideration would need to be given to Lionel's difficulties around eating and food preparation. It may be necessary to discuss treatment options with Lionel and I suggest a psychologist's assessment in order to facilitate a residential placement.

HO 19b: Lionel Jenkins: The 'short and sweet' version

Current situation

Lionel Jenkins is 82-years-old, lives alone and has been supported by his daughter, Dorothy for the last ten years. He has a congestive heart condition. Dorothy has helped him with personal care and domestic tasks, but she has been diagnosed with liver cancer and is now unable to look after her father. Lionel has a son, but Lionel does not want to live with him. Lionel has for the last 20 years been unable to eat or drink in front of anyone else, including his daughter. He insists that she wear a mask while preparing his food. Lionel now wants to return to Swansea and move into residential care.

Background information

Lionel was born in Swansea. He married and two children were adopted. Lionel's wife died in 1981. He remarried 18 months after his wife's death. His second wife left him in 1993. He believes this was partly due to his not being able to eat in front of other people. On his daughter's advice, he moved to Bristol in 1994.

Immediate needs

Lionel requires immediate support in relation to washing, dressing, shopping, food preparation and cleaning, while he continues to live in Bristol. Home Care would be the most appropriate option, although staff would need to be aware of Lionel's difficulties in relation to eating, drinking and food preparation.

In the meantime residential care options in Swansea will need to be investigated. Consideration would again have to be given to Lionel's difficulties around eating and food preparation. Further treatment options may need to be discussed with Lionel and a psychologist's assessment recommended, in order to facilitate a residential placement. At the moment he is reluctant to consider this.

HO 19c: Lionel Jenkins: The 'does the job' version

Current situation

Lionel Jenkins is 82-years-old, living on his own in Bristol, where he has been supported by his daughter Dorothy. He has a congestive heart condition, which leaves him exhausted after any activity. Dorothy has helped him to wash and dress as well as shopping, preparing food and cleaning. Dorothy has recently been diagnosed with liver cancer and is no longer able to look after her father. Lionel has a son, Harold, but Lionel does not want to live with him. Lionel has, for the last 20 years, been unable to eat or drink in front of anyone else, including his daughter. He has also insisted that Dorothy wear a mask while preparing his food. Lionel now wants to return to his hometown Swansea and move into residential care.

Background information

Lionel was born in Swansea, the eldest of eight children. He described his mother as a strong character and he was her favourite. He developed TB when he was 17, and then spent most of World War II in hospital or convalescing. It was at this time he met his future wife, Pearl. He says that due to the tensions caused by his mother's dislike of Pearl and his frustration at not being able to serve during the war, he suffered a 'nervous collapse'. He was in hospital for six months. After his discharge he married Pearl, and his mother accepted the situation. As they were unable to have children, Lionel and Pearl adopted Dorothy and Harold. Lionel says there were always problems with Harold, which later put Lionel and his wife under financial pressure as they tried to help him over the years.

Lionel feels it was the worry over Harold which led to his wife's death in 1981. Eighteen months later he married Brenda, who had been a friend to the couple and had helped nurse Pearl when she was dying of breast cancer. Shortly after this his mother died. Despite the problems between them, he had always had a very strong relationship with his mother and he missed her a great deal. Lionel says that it was then that he began to have problems eating in front of people. He says that he finds it difficult to swallow. He didn't mind eating in front of Brenda, but not anyone else. Lionel says that Brenda encouraged him to get help, but he didn't want to see anyone about it. She stayed for ten years, but in the end she got fed up and she left him in 1993.

Lionel then lived on his own for a year, and found it increasingly difficult to cope. On his daughter's advice, he moved to a small flat, close to Dorothy in Bristol in 1994. Even though he didn't leave a large number of friends, Lionel says he found the move a 'terrible upheaval'.

Immediate needs

Although Lionel has not discussed Dorothy's long term prognosis with her, he knows that she is unable to look after him anymore. He says he dreads being on his own and has decided to move into residential care in Swansea, so that he can 'end his days in his hometown'. He believes this will reassure Dorothy to know that he is alright. Lionel says that he accepts there is little that can be done for his heart condition and that he is just 'grateful for whatever time he has left'.

Lionel says he is particular about where he goes in Swansea and wants to avoid the 'rough' parts of the city. He would also like to be able to take some of his own things, including his bed and his chair. Lionel says that he owns his own flat, which he thinks is worth about £130,000, and that he still has about £20,000 in savings and investments. He receives a pension from the bank on top of his state pension, as well as claiming attendance allowance. Lionel says he wants help finding a home in Swansea. He knows that he will have to make a contribution to the cost.

Lionel requires immediate support in relation to washing, dressing, shopping, food preparation and cleaning. Home Care would be the most appropriate option, although staff would need to be aware of Lionel's difficulties in relation to eating, drinking and food preparation.

In the meantime residential care options in Swansea can be explored. Lionel is concerned that people should understand his particular needs around eating and drinking. He says it is important for them to respect his problems and that he really could not eat anything unless it had been prepared according to his requirements. When this was pointed out as a potential area of difficulty, especially in a communal residential setting, Lionel said that he would have to insist his conditions were met. I suggested that it might be helpful if Lionel spoke to a psychologist, who might be able to help him. Lionel was reluctant to pursue this. It may be necessary to discuss this option further with Lionel in order to address the problems, which might otherwise restrict the residential placements available.

Section B: It's obvious isn't it?

✓ Exercise 10: What else do you need to know?

↗ Objective

To identify how recordings may make assumptions, which do not make clear the basis on which an opinion has been reached or a decision has been made.

🕐 Timing

Allow 1 hour for this exercise.

✏ Materials

- HO 20: What else do you need to know?
- Pens and paper
- Flipchart stand and paper
- OHP
- OHT 10: What else do you need to know?

ⓘ Trainer's guidelines

Step 1: allow 5 minutes.
Show OHT 10 and explain the problems arising from case recording, which assumes the reader will understand issues which have not been clearly explained in the record.

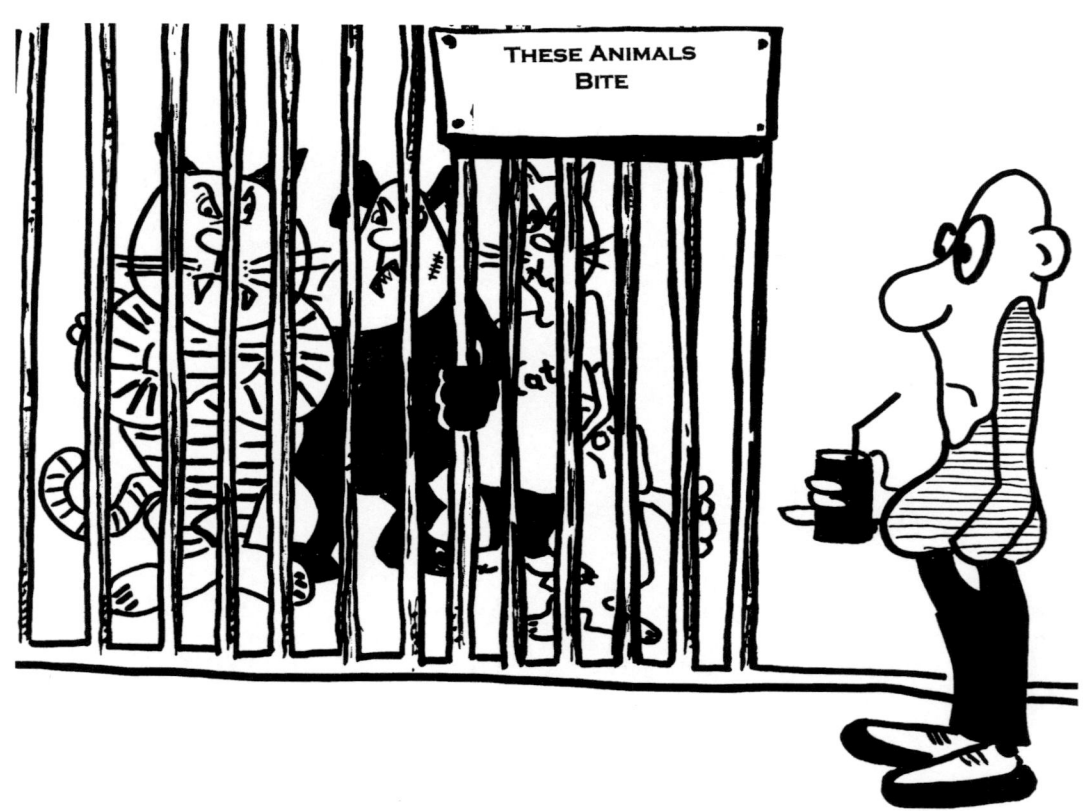

Step 2: allow 5 minutes.
Give out HO 20: What else do you need to know? Divide the participants into groups of three or four. Ask them to discuss the examples on the sheet and identify what questions the reader is left asking, and what information should be included to make an effective record.

Step 3: allow 30 minutes
Participants work through the case sheet

Step 4: allow 20 minutes.
Ask participants to return to the main group, while still remaining with their small groups. Review each statement on the case sheet. Ask the small groups in turn for their response to each statement. Let one group provide the main feedback for a particular statement, and then ask the other groups if they have anything further they want to say. Move on to the next group to provide the main feedback for the next statement, and so on until all the statements have been discussed.

OHT 10: What else do you need to know?

Identified problems with case recording:

- There is a lack of evidence for the decisions made.

How do you decide what information needs to be included?

Has the reader enough information to understand:

- The basis on which a decision has been made?

- The basis on which an opinion has been formed?

- The significance of how a situation has been described?

- The significance of what is recorded for the department's role in relation to the service user?

HO 20: What else do you need to know?

Identify how this information is inadequate and what questions the reader is left asking. Assume that the recording is part of an ongoing case file, but that this particular entry has been made without any further details:

Example 1

• The situation is now stable. No further action required.

Example 2

• Spoken with Mr Jones. All avenues of support have been explored, but he is resolute in his refusal to accept any more help.

Example 3

• Spoken with GP this morning, and he thinks there is little point in Mrs D attending the alcohol treatment programme, given what has happened before.

Example 4

• Mrs S said she was 'at the end of her tether' when I spoke with her this morning, and felt that her husband had become 'more impossible' since his stroke. I suggested a carer's assessment should be made.

Example 5

• Mr W phoned the office today to complain about his home carer. I asked if he wanted to make a formal complaint and he said no, so I said I would have a word with the home care organiser.

Example 6

• Ronnie said he was fed up with attending the resource centre and wanted to get a real job. Staff at the centre said they thought Ronnie was unrealistic in his expectations. I told Ronnie that he needed to concentrate on his IT skills first.

Example 7

• Spoke with warden from sheltered housing unit. She said Mrs Y was becoming too difficult, and the other residents thought she was a nuisance. It seems Mrs Y's confusion is getting worse. Mrs Y's daughter does not want her mother to go into residential care yet, and Mrs Y is adamant she wants to stay in her own place.

Example 8

• Mr K said he is not taking his medication, as he does not like the side effects.

Example 9

- Ms O is unlikely to benefit from further intervention.

Example 10

- Bernard's mother feels this is an inappropriate placement for Bernard as he needs a higher level of support.

Exercise 11: Filling in the gaps

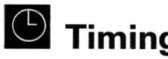 **Objective**

To identify how recordings may only tell part of the story, leaving the reader to fill in the gaps with their own assumptions.

Timing

Allow 45 minutes for this exercise

Materials

- HO 21: Filling in the gaps
- Pens and paper
- Flipchart stand or white-board

Trainer's guidelines

Step 1: allow 5 minutes
Divide participants into groups of between three and four members. Give them the HO 21: Filling in the gaps and ask them to read the scenario.

Step 2: allow 20 minutes
Ask participants to identify where the record is insufficient in the information it provides. What questions are left unanswered?

Step 3: allow 20 minutes
Ask participants to return to the larger group, seated still with their small group. Ask each group in turn to identify a particular deficiency in the record. Continue going round the groups until all the points are exhausted.

Compare with the 'Trainer Notes' and add any remaining points.

☐ HO 21: Filling in the gaps: Camila Fernandez

Background information

Camila Fernandez is a 24-year-old woman with a mild learning disability, who has recently moved into a small group home, living with three other people and supported by staff who visit the home daily for two hours.

Camila's parents came to Britain from Chile in the 1970s. Her mother and father separated 12 years ago and he returned to Chile. Her mother died six months ago which prompted Camila's move into the group home. Camila was adamant she did not want to leave Britain and her father said he did not feel there were suitable facilities to support her living in Chile.

Record of visit to Camila Fernandez by social worker

Responding to a request to visit Camila because she has been feeling increasingly unhappy in the group home. Staff have reported tensions between the residents.

Camila said that, although she had first liked the home and the other people living there, she had become increasingly miserable over the last few months. We discussed the reasons for this and her feelings towards the other residents, as well as her feelings about her mother's death, which is still fairly recent.

It was clear that she has found adjusting to a group living situation rather difficult and has become somewhat isolated, despite the staff's attempts to support her through the grieving process, and integrate her with the other residents.

Camila said she was still attending the resource centre, and we discussed how she had been getting on with the cookery classes she had been attending. It seemed that Camila felt more positive about the time she spent at the centre.

She said she had received a letter from her father in the last month in which he said he wished he could do more to help her. Camila talked about her memories of her father before he returned to Chile.

Camila said that, as she did not like the other people living in the home, she did not want to stay there. I explained that finding another home might take some time and so she would not be able to move immediately. I suggested that in the meantime, I could visit her more regularly to discuss the problems she was having.

Trainer notes

1. Who has requested the visit?
2. What is meant by unhappy? Who has described Camila as unhappy?
3. What is meant by 'tensions'? Who has used this term?
4. What is meant by 'few months'? How long has Camila been feeling miserable?
5. What reasons did Camila give for feeling miserable?
6. What does Camila feel about the other residents and why?
7. How is she feeling about her mother's death?
8. In what ways has she found adjusting to group living difficult?
9. What examples are provided of these difficulties?
10. What form does her isolation take?
11. What attempts have been made by the staff to integrate her with the other residents?
12. What attempts have they made to support her in the grieving process?
13. How does Camila feel about the staff?
14. What progress has she made with the cookery class?
15. Why does she feel more positive about the resource centre and what evidence is there of this?
16. What did she say about her father and her memories of him?
17. What problems is the social worker proposing to discuss and to what purpose; support and/or trying to resolve them?

Chapter 4: I'd Like to Tell You But . . .

Section A: Introduction: How comfortable are we to share information with service users?

Best practice is based on key principles of partnership, openness and accuracy. Effective recording is part of the total service to the user. Social service departments need to give clear guidance and training which promotes working in partnership with service users and carers. This includes constructing and sharing written records.

Department of Health, Data Protection Act 1998,
Guidance to Social Services, S3.2

Let's remind ourselves briefly why we record people's personal information [as detailed in *For the Record: Recording Skills Training Manual* (Liz O'Rourke, 2002)]:

- Accountability: to explain, justify or challenge in the future, the service decisions we make that can make a big impact on the lives of service users; to fulfil legal requirements, e.g. looked after children, mental health, audit, data protection.
- To communicate between care workers, so ensuring continuity and consistency of care for the service user.

Both of these put the service user centre stage. But the information we gather isn't always straightforward . . .

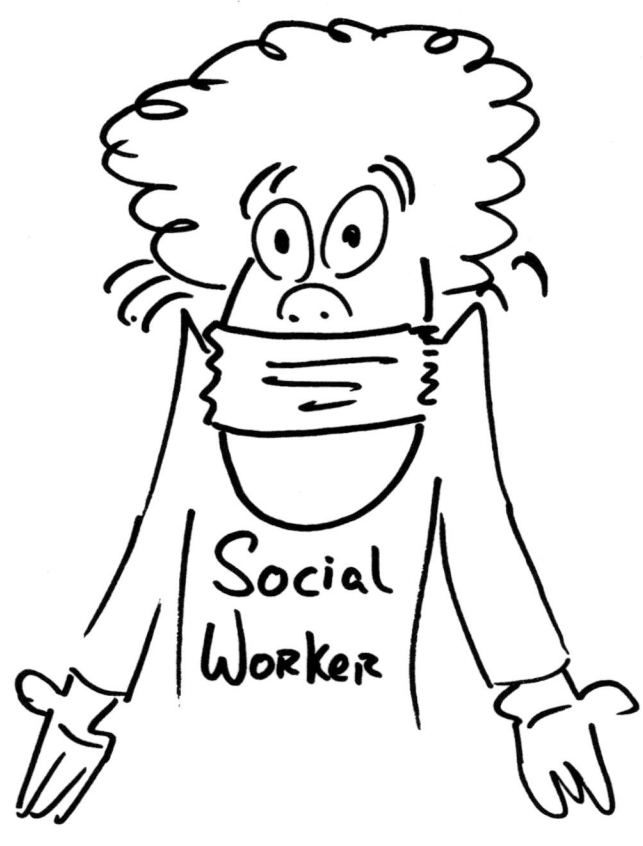

✔️ Exercise 12: Open recording is an ideal, but how easy is it in reality?

↗️ Objective

To explore the obstacles that complicate open recording

🕐 Timing

Allow 30 minutes for this exercise

✏️ Materials

- HO 22: Checklist exercise
- HO 23: Openness is the ideal but can it always be unlimited?
- Individual, large font masters of Exercise 12
- Flipchart and marker pens
- Post-its
- Pens

ⓘ Trainer's guidelines

Step 1: allow 5 minutes
Give out HO 22 as you explain that this is a quick, checklist exercise to be completed individually. Ask participants to tick those questions they've encountered when recording their work with service users.

Step 2: allow 15 minutes
After participants have completed step 1, arrange the masters of each question around the room/on the wall. Then ask participants to share with their neighbour (or neighbours if an odd number) which of those they ticked they found most difficult, and the reasons why, and then to write these on post-its.

Step 3: allow 10 minutes
Ask participants to attach their completed post-its to the master list of questions (on the wall) and to consider each other's contributions. This can take the form of a review discussion led by the trainer.

Step 4
Give out HO 23: Openness is the ideal but can it always be unlimited?

▣ HO 22: Checklist exercise: Open recording is the ideal, but how easy is it in reality?

Step 1: 5 minutes
Tick each of the dilemmas below that you've encountered when trying to record details about a service user:

1.   Are the facts unclear, inconsistent or confused?
2.   Do family members disagree with each other?
3.   Do all agencies and professionals agree on the facts and opinions?
4.   Has the service user, their carer or family told you something they've asked you not to tell the others?
5.   Has another agency or professional given you information they say you can't share with the service user or their family?
6.   Does the fact that you've been asked *not* to share certain information affect the options you can discuss with the service user?
7.   Have you been given information you're not sure is relevant or reliable?
8.   Do you always record everything you are told?
9.   Is information embarrassing? To whom?
10. Do the service user's view and yours sometimes conflict?

Step 2: 15 minutes
Share with your neighbour (or neighbours) which of those you ticked you found most difficult and the reasons why, and write these on post-its.

Step 3: 10 minutes
Attach your completed post-its to the master list of questions (on the wall) and look at each other's contributions.

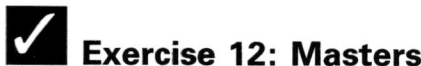 **Exercise 12: Masters**

Are the facts unclear, inconsistent or confused?

Do family members disagree with each other?

Do all agencies and professionals agree on the facts and opinions?

Has the service user, their carer or family told you something they've asked you not to tell the others?

Has another agency or professional given you information they say you can't share with the service user or their family?

Does the fact that you've been asked not to share certain information affect the options you can discuss with the service user?

Have you been given information you're not sure is relevant or reliable?

Do you always record everything you are told?

Is information embarrassing? To whom?

Do the service user's view and yours sometimes conflict?

📄 HO 23: Openness is the ideal, but can it always be unlimited?

Staff in public service and the caring professions have a duty of confidence to those they serve, and to those from whom they seek and obtain information. People have a right to privacy,[1] and the more sensitive their details, the more privacy is essential. People also have a right to their health and safety being safeguarded. One person's privacy might conflict with another's right to proper measures for their health and safety being taken,[2] for instance:

> *In 1993, Essex CC placed a 15-year-old boy with regular foster carers, the 'W' family, without telling them of his history of sexual abuse. In the month the boy was with the family, he sexually abused all four of the foster parents' own children, aged 8–12. The children were traumatised, the parents' marriage collapsed and the father was off work long-term with post-traumatic stress. Ten years later, the family was awarded £190,000 in an out-of-court settlement.[3]*

Telling the foster carers about the most sensitive aspects of the boy's history would have denied his right to privacy. But not doing so failed to meet their right to safeguard their health and safety, and their right to family life.

Having information can sometimes cause distress, even damage:

- Someone is terminally ill, but the doctors and family have decided they would be badly affected by knowing that, to the detriment of their physical and mental health.
- A woman tells social services in strictest confidence that she is extremely concerned about the way her neighbours are treating their child. If the neighbours knew she had told social services, there could be unfortunate consequences for her, the child and the investigation.

In some circumstances, the law can prevent information being made available:

- A resident of a home for elderly people confides in her relatives that one of the staff regularly steals money from her handbag. While the member of staff accused has a right to defend themselves from such allegations, the police might need to investigate how many other possible victims there are, so the named member of staff won't necessarily know anything about the accusation at first. A young person is found guilty of an offence in court. Their name can't be routinely published, to safeguard a vulnerable, immature person.

The law also says that personal information held for social work purposes[4] need not be shared with the person concerned if that is likely to cause serious harm to someone: the person concerned or someone else.

In other circumstances, the law insists on information being made available:

---

[1] Human Rights Act 1998, Article 8: '1. Everyone has the right to respect for his [*sic*] private and family life, his home and his correspondence. 2. There shall be no interference by a public authority with the exercise of this right except such as is in accordance with the law and is necessary in a democratic society in the interests of national security, public safety or the economic well-being of the country, for the prevention of disorder or crime, for the protection of health or morals, or for the protection of the rights and freedoms of others.'

[2] There is a further relevant right under the Human Rights Act 1998, Article 3: 'No one shall be subjected to torture or to inhuman or degrading treatment or punishment.'

[3] BBC News, 2nd January 2002: http://news.bbc.co.uk/1/england/1738344.stm

[4] The Data Protection (Subject Access Modification) (Social Work) Order 2000.

- Official enquiries, such as the Laming enquiry into the death of Victoria Climbié and the Bichard enquiry into how the agencies handled information about Ian Huntley, require the detailed publication of personal information because it cannot now harm the victims, but is clearly in the public interest to publish: doing so might increase understanding and help avoid similar tragedies in the future.

And for that matter, how many of us know someone socially whose personal hygiene gives us a problem, and we find it impossible to tell them? But not telling them means that they continue being socially tagged as 'smelly' without the chance to address the problem. And anyway, who's to say it's their problem rather than ours?

Whether to give information, or not to give information, can be complicated – and clearly very important.

✓ Exercise 13: What you can and can't share

↗ Objective

1. To explore what information you can and can't share, and why.
2. To use difficulties faced today with yesterday's recording to help avoid tomorrow's problems.

🕐 Timing

Allow 1 hour for this exercise

✏️ Materials

- HO 24: What you can and can't share
- Flipchart paper and marker pens
- Blu tack or masking tape

ℹ️ Trainer's guidelines

Step 1: allow 30 minutes
Divide participants into groups of four (approximately, depending on number of participants). Give out HO 24 and ask them:

1. To read each of the four following scenarios (5 minutes).
2. Agree someone to act as scribe, someone to report back later to the full group.
3. Then identify on flipchart paper the recording issues they think each poses (15 minutes).

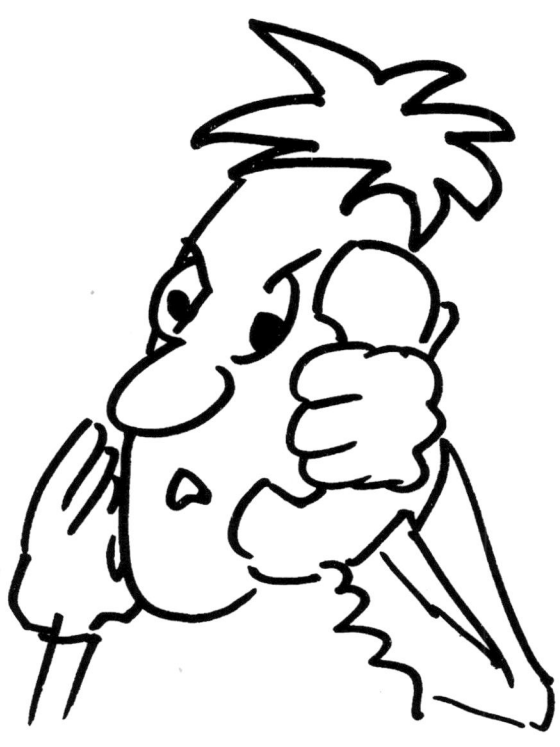

4.   Identify what might be done differently in each case, to overcome the information difficulty (10 minutes).

Step 2: allow 20 minutes
Ask each sub-group to put their flipchart page on the wall/board in turn and explain their findings to the large group.

Step 3: allow 10 minutes
Discuss the key lessons about involving the people whose information we record. How far are they practice issues, how far recording issues?

It would be useful at the end of this session to give participants the SSI's 1997 Inspection Standards on case records. Draw attention in particular to Standards 1.3; 1.4; 1.5; 1.6; 1.9; 1.10; 2.2; 2.6; 4.1; 4.3; 4.4; 4.5; 4.6; 4.7.
[www.dh.gov.uk/assetRoot/04/03/56/80/04035680.pdf]

▣ HO 24: **What you can and can't share**

Step 1: 30 minutes total

1. In small groups, read each of the four following scenarios (5 minutes).
2. Agree someone to act as scribe, someone to report back later to the full group.
3. Then identify on flipchart paper the recording issues each poses (15 minutes).
4. Identify what might be done differently in each case, to overcome the information difficulty (10 minutes).

Scenario 1: Mrs Edith Norman and Mrs Pauline Brent

Mrs Norman is an 87-year-old white woman. She had a stroke two years ago which left her left side paralysed. After leaving hospital, she went to live with her daughter, Mrs Brent. The social services department provided equipment and continues to provide domiciliary care for key periods while Mrs Brent is out at work. Mrs Brent's husband left her a year ago, following disagreements about Mrs Norman continuing to live with them. Mrs Brent is a teacher who plans to retire in a year's time. She has recently been advised by her doctor that she has high blood pressure.

Mrs Brent's GP (who is also Mrs Norman's) has asked for help for Mrs Brent in her care of Mrs Norman. During a meeting between yourself and Mrs Brent, she becomes distressed and tearful. She says she's desperate for her mother to leave, but can't say so to her; that her mother becomes distressed when she has started to broach the possibility. She says she wants her mother to go into a home, but asks you not to tell her she said so. She believes that her blood pressure results from caring for her mother, and that her relationship with her husband could be repaired if Mrs Norman were no longer there. The prospect of retiring in a year's time to full-time care of her mother, and losing the outlets that her job currently provides, she finds unendurable. She asks you to persuade Mrs Norman to consider residential care, and to tell her mother that you and the GP think it's the best thing.

Mrs Norman is also distressed when talking to you: about the stroke and her consequent dependency, losing her husband (Mrs Brent's stepfather) three years ago, the loss of her house, and at her daughter's hinting at her going into a home, which she dreads. She thinks her daughter is better off without Mr Brent, whom she thinks weak and selfish. She never got on with him, just as Mrs Brent never got on with her stepfather, Mrs Norman's second husband. She says that, with the services she gets, and with all the mod cons of a modern kitchen, her daughter hasn't that much to do for her physically. Her blood pressure would be sorted if she retired a bit earlier than next year: she's already worked 30 years as a teacher, she'd get a good pension.

Scenario 2: James Barratt

Mr Barratt is a 79-year-old white man. He's suffered for some years with respiratory and heart disease, and now has inoperable cancer. He's very frail and dependent on oxygen and drugs to manage his pain. You've been asked to re-assess his social care needs in preparation for his leaving hospital. Mr Barratt knows how ill he is, and is very anxious to go home for his remaining time. His wife died 12 years ago, but his daughter and son-in-law live just a few doors away and offer him daily help with shopping, cooking and washing. You read his social services records. They refer to his conviction 25 years ago for sexually abusing the 15-year-old girl who then lived next door.

Scenario 3: Jenny Stevenson

Jenny is a 23-year-old white woman with learning disabilities. She lives in a supported flat. Recently, with the help of an advocate, Jenny has asked to see the records of her time in the care of the authority. She wants to understand why she was removed from the Lawrences, her foster carers, to residential school. Martin and Annette Lawrence were foster parents for some years, but withdrew from fostering after Jenny's placement ended. You look over the records dating back eight years, and find the Lawrences quoted as claiming that Jenny was sexually provocative and aggressive, and stole money from them. They are also quoted as saying that they felt the department gave them very little help at the time. It's not clear from the record how far any of this was discussed with Jenny, nor whether the Lawrences believed this was confidential between themselves and their social worker.

Scenario 4: Mrs Margaret Fraser

Denise March is a newly appointed social worker in a hospital-based team. She's asked to visit Mrs Fraser to assess her social care needs prior to leaving hospital. On arriving on the ward, the nurse directs her to the medical files in the office, where Denise reads that Mrs Fraser has Motor Neurone Disease. When she introduces herself to Mrs Fraser, she realises it's not clear how much Mrs Fraser is aware of her condition herself. Her husband is urging her to come home, he's finding it difficult to cope with work and looking after the home. He seems unaware of his wife's condition. Mrs Fraser's conversation consists mainly of her worries about her husband not being able to cope alone at home. She also expresses the hope the doctors will be able to get her back on her feet again.

Step 2: 20 minutes
In the full group, each sub-group shows their flipchart page on the wall/board in turn and explains their findings to the large group.

Step 3: 10 minutes
The full group to discuss the key lessons about involving the people whose information we record. How far are they practice issues, how far recording issues?

Trainer notes

Scenario 1: Mrs Edith Norman and Mrs Pauline Brent

Should you write one or separate assessments?

- The needs of both women are interwoven. If you write separate assessments, how will you reconcile their different needs and wishes? But you've got confidential information you can't share.
- You could share with Mrs Brent and Mrs Norman the kind of assessment(s) you'd have to write if they won't share their difficult feelings and wishes with each other, and ask them how effective they think that would be.
- You could help them explore how they think the other would respond, if their assessments were written and shared in these less than open terms.
- You could help them find ways of expressing to each other their real feelings and wishes in ways they could feel comfortable with. This might take more time than the pressure of work might easily allow, but in the long run, be more effective. Negotiating what to say or write encourages clarity of thought, and engages and empowers people.

Scenario 2: Mr James Barratt

Why is this 25 year old information on the file?

- It's sensitive information. Might be justified. But is it relevant to today's circumstances? Does the file explain the offence and conviction further? This might be a case of a record holding both too much and too little information: enough fact to cause anxiety, not enough context so you can assess its relevance now.

Is there any current risk to anyone?

- Mr Barratt is almost certainly too ill and frail to be a risk to anyone, and there is no information to suggest there had been more recent concerns.

- This could unnecessarily colour how others see Mr Barratt, others he needs help from.

Scenario 3: Jenny Stevenson

What (if any) information can foster carers expect to be confidential from the children they care for? Is their consent necessary to share this with Jenny?

- In fact, people are generally entitled to the information provided by foster carers, like social care workers, unless there are exceptional reasons such as the likelihood of harm to someone, including the person it's about. But it's possible that hasn't in the past been clear to foster carers.

If it's possible that Jenny might not know what was said about her then, being told now after all these years might be very distressing:

- A balance should be struck between: Jenny's right to information about herself; and the risk of harm to herself or others if the information distressed or angered her. The worker could do a risk assessment:[5] what are the risks, and to whom, of telling Jenny, or not telling Jenny?

- She has an advocate. The social services department might not have carried out its duty of care to Jenny well enough in the past. By giving her the information now she has the chance to pursue redress. The department could, together with the advocate, give Jenny support now to deal with that information.

How might we record the information if this happened today?

Scenario 4: Mrs Margaret Fraser

Would social workers usually read the medical notes at the invitation of the nurse, before seeing the service user?

- The problem is that Denise now has information without knowing if Mrs Fraser also has it, so has to tread warily. This rather restricts her ability to discuss Mrs Fraser's circumstances and needs with her, and how to meet them.
- You need the explicit consent[6] of the person concerned to let someone from another agency or profession have their medical information. Good practice would suggest that Denise visits Mrs Fraser and asks her what she needs to know. Denise isn't a medical professional, so even if she read the medical notes with Mrs Fraser's consent, she isn't professionally competent to interpret them. If, after speaking to Mrs Fraser, Denise still needs clarification about the effect of her medical condition on Mrs Fraser's social care needs, assessment and recording would be more straightforward if she asked Mrs Fraser if it was OK to check with the medical staff. She could then check exactly what they had told Mrs Fraser and her husband.
- Does the hospital make medical notes routinely available to patients? Is there a difference between those they might keep in the office, and those available to patients? Which if any does Denise (need to) have access to?
- Does the hospital know how Denise would use the medical records?

As the single, shared or unified assessment Process develops further, the need for consent to share information with other agencies remains just as necessary, as do the additional requirements for sharing sensitive information (such as health information); but what has changed is the point at which consent needs to be obtained in order to assemble and share assessment information at the outset.

---

[5] See Risk assessment in relation to recording and sharing information, HO 31.
[6] Data Protection Act 1998, S2 and Sch 3.

Section B: Open and above board

Inclusive recording means using respectful language which is not oppressive. What we record reveals a lot about how we work with service users: do we see them as passive, detached objects to be observed and commented upon, or as active partners in a collaborative process? Conventional case recording has tended to be of the former variety. Conventional recording also allows the writer's own values and subjective perceptions to enter unchallenged or unnoticed.

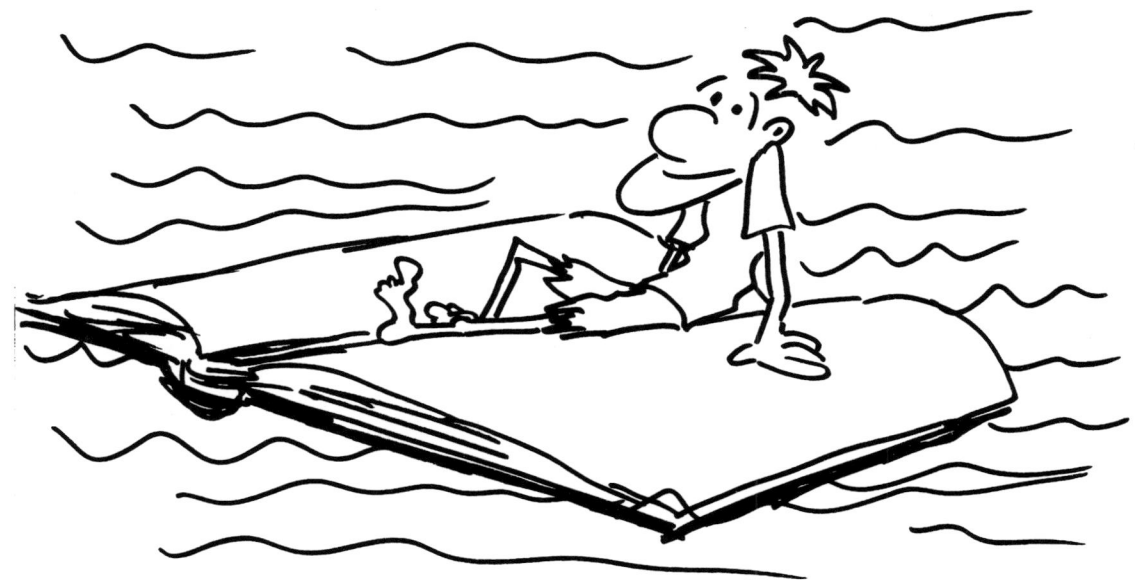

✓ **Exercise 14: Inclusive recording**

↗ **Objectives**

1. To explore how records might be written in a more inclusive way.
2. To explore the insidious and powerful use of language.

🕐 **Timing**

Allow 30 minutes for this exercise (40 if using the optional third step).

✎ **Materials**

*   HO 25: Inclusive recording
*   Pens
*   OHP and OHT 11: Inclusive recording
*   OHP pen

ⓘ **Trainer's guidelines**

Step 1: allow 15 minutes
Divide participants into groups of four (depending on number of participants). Give out HO 25: ask them to consider each of the case extracts and discuss what they consider oppressive. Ask them to underline words and phrases they think fit that description. Suggest some questions to ask themselves. These might include 'How would I feel if this was written about me/my family?', 'What would a lawyer make of this?', 'What impression does it give me of someone I've not yet met?'

Step 2: allow 15 minutes
Bring participants back to the full group. Invite participants to share what they have discovered. You could use the questions above to start the discussion. Underline the words and phrases they noted as oppressive on the OHT 11. Ask them why they identified these.

Step 3: (optional) allow 10 minutes
Ask participants to rewrite one scenario of their choosing, avoiding oppressive language, basing it on the evidence available.

▣ HO 25: Inclusive recording

Step 1: 15 minutes

1. Read each of the following extracts (5 minutes).
2. Discuss in your group what might be considered oppressive, underlining words and phrases you think fit that description (10 minutes).

(Questions might include 'How would I feel if this was written about me?', 'What would a lawyer make of this?', 'What impression does it give me of someone I've not yet met?')

Case file extracts

1. Mrs Woolgar seemed more depressed on this occasion. Relationship with husband still tense. The flat was dirty and untidy. They both continue to blame social services for all their problems. Probable displacement of the unresolved issues in their relationship.
2. Mr Patel is clearly a very devout man who accepts his present circumstances with a fatalistic resignation. He is always polite and courteous, although he does not believe there is anything anyone can do to change his situation.
3. When Mr Guthrie arrived, he was obviously in a combative mood. He made it clear that he thought the review was a waste of time. He hurled abuse at everyone, complaining that none of us cared about what happened to him or his wife.
4. Mrs Hemmings is increasingly manipulative in her attitude. She seems to go along with what I say, but I don't feel she has any real intention of co-operating. Her neighbour said she had been arguing with her over the dog barking.
5. Mrs Wheeler presents as a very capable and well-organised woman. She is determined to maintain her independence and seems unwilling to acknowledge the restrictions her increasing disability will place on her. This denial may be a coping reaction to her illness.

Step 2: 15 minutes
Return to the main group to share your views. You could use these questions as a start:

1. How would I feel if this was written about me?
2. What would a lawyer make of this?
3. What impression does it give me of someone I've not yet met?
4. What words and phrases do I find oppressive, and why?

Step 3: (optional) – allow 10 minutes
Rewrite one scenario, avoiding oppressive language, basing it on the evidence available.

OHT 11: Inclusive recording

1. Mrs Woolgar seemed more depressed on this occasion. Relationship with husband still tense. The flat was dirty and untidy. They both continue to blame social services for all their problems. Probable displacement of the unresolved issues in their relationship.

2. Mr Patel is clearly a very devout man who accepts his present circumstances with a fatalistic resignation. He is always polite and courteous, although he does not believe there is anything anyone can do to change his situation.

3. When Mr Guthrie arrived, he was obviously in a combative mood. He made it clear that he thought the review was a waste of time. He hurled abuse at everyone, complaining that none of us cared about what happened to him or his wife.

4. Mrs Hemmings is increasingly manipulative in her attitude. She seems to go along with what I say, but I don't feel she has any real intention of co-operating. Her neighbour said she had been arguing with her over the dog barking.

5. Mrs Wheeler presents as a very capable and well-organised woman. She is determined to maintain her independence and seems unwilling to acknowledge the restrictions her increasing disability will place on her. This denial may be a coping reaction to her illness.

Trainer notes

Different groups of participants will mark different words and phrases, and it would be possible to identify most for one reason or another, for example:

1. Mrs Woolgar

Mrs Woolgar **seemed** more **depressed** on this occasion. Relationship with husband **still tense**. The flat was **dirty and untidy**. They **both continue** to blame the department for **all their problems**. **Probable displacement** of the **unresolved** issues in their relationship.

- **Seemed**: allows the writer to convey a fact or impression without evidence or commitment.
- **Depressed**: a word that conveys a wide spectrum of mood, not qualified here
- **Still**: conveys ongoing tension, but with no timescale, leaves the reader to imagine how long.
- **Tense**: no specifics, the reader is left to imagine. Arrests attention, focuses on the person, not on why. 'Why' might be understandable.
- **Dirty and untidy**: subjective and relative adjectives, no detail. But together, they double the impact.
- **Both**: 'both' is unnecessary, but reinforces 'they', conveys alliance, collusion.
- **Continue**: they've not just blamed the department once, but 'continue' to do so. Department mightn't have responded effectively, but with no explanation, conveys unreasonableness, uncooperativeness.
- **All their problems**: how many problems, or how severe unclear; but 'all' conveys many, and failure of personal responsibility for 'all their problems'.
- **Probable**: word that's safe to use when not sure of facts or opinion; still conveys message that a thing is so, without being accountable for it.
- **Displacement**: a psychoanalytical term, and such technical words give credibility to the person using them, though not necessarily deserved!
- **Unresolved**: whether the couple have unresolved problems in their relationship, or whether they are frustrated at the department's ineffectual or unreliable involvement, there is no evidence to indicate either way.

2. Mr Patel

Mr Patel is **clearly** a **very** devout man who **accepts** his present circumstances with a **fatalistic resignation**. He is **always** polite and courteous, although he does not believe there is anything anyone can do to change his situation.

- **Clearly**: conveys certainty, unnecessary if evidence supports the claim.
- **Very**: devout means 'deeply religious', so **very** an unnecessary emphasis.
- **Accepts/fatalistic resignation**: accepts on its own can convey 'sees favourably' or 'approves', 'believes to be correct'; as well as 'submits to'; but together with **fatalistic resignation**, they convey an impression of passivity or hopelessness. **Fatalistic resignation** might equally be based on a lack of knowledge or understanding of Mr Patel's religious beliefs.

- **Always**: consistently having a positive attribute (always polite) is a positive description – but in the context of the overall description, it can sound like a negative attribute, conveying a lack of discernment, energy or purpose.

3. Mr Guthrie

When Mr Guthrie arrived, he was **obviously** in a **combative mood**. He **made it clear** that he thought the review was **a waste of time**. He **hurled abuse** at everyone, **complaining** that none of us cared about what happened to him or his wife.

- **Obviously**: like **clearly** above (2, Mr Patel), conveys certainty, unnecessary if evidence supports the claim.
- **Combative mood**: **combative** means fighting, belligerent, bellicose, conveying physical aggression. But **mood** suggests Mr Guthrie isn't actually threatening physical violence. Angry, cross, annoyed, irritated . . . for lack of further evidence, one person's 'combative' is another person's 'irritated'. A word meaning 'fighting' being coupled with 'mood', however, is a double whammy: 'being in a mood' is always associated with a 'bad' rather than a 'good' mood.
- **Made it clear**: did he just say what he wanted unambiguously, or did he repeat it, or did he shout it, or did he loom over the person to whom he was making it clear . . . without context, again it's for every reader's interpretation.
- **Waste of time**: direct quote or writer's interpretation? Together with the other underlined words, builds up a picture of aggression and a totally rejecting attitude. That might be the case, but the picture is a vivid one lacking specific evidence to back the description up. What exactly did he do to earn the descriptions?
- **Hurled abuse**: reinforces the 'combative mood' picture. 'Hurling abuse' leaves to the reader's imagination what Mr Guthrie said, and that might be quite mild on the reader's own scale of what 'hurling abuse' means.
- **Complaining**: tends to be seen as negative, at least when others do it to us!

4. Mrs Hemmings

Mrs Hemmings is **increasingly manipulative in her attitude**. She **seems** to **go along with what I say**, but **I don't feel she has any real intention** of co-operating. **Her neighbour said** she had been **arguing** with her over the dog barking.

- **Increasingly**: indicates history; together with 'manipulative', a negative one.
- **Manipulative in her attitude**: a negative word, yet it lacks specifics. As the description continues, a vivid picture is constructed without substance.
- **Seems**: as with Mrs Woolgar (1) allows the writer to convey a fact or impression without evidence or commitment.
- **Go along with what I say**: continued from 'manipulative in her attitude', there is as much evidence for the worker's failure to listen to and engage with Mrs Hemmings, who might be too polite or feeling too disempowered to disagree with her.

- **I don't feel**: used as a less committed substitute for 'in my opinion', or 'I think' or 'I believe'. 'Feel' lets the writer express an opinion whilst still having a let out if proved wrong, letting the writer have it both ways.
- **She has (not) any real intention**: continues the picture of Mrs Hemmings being responsible for the failure of the worker's involvement.
- **Her neighbour said**: the first and only quote, indirect though it is, isn't from Mrs Hemmings, the central character, but from her neighbour.
- **Arguing**: the neighbour's perception. The dog might have been alone and barking all day; it might have been barking at night, early in the morning, or every time a car passed. Mrs Hemmings might just have asked politely if they could restrain it, and the neighbour, as is human nature, might be overreacting defensively. We don't know without more details: Mrs Hemmings' version is absent.

5. Mrs Wheeler

Mrs Wheeler **presents** as a **very** capable and well-organised woman. She is **determined** to maintain her independence and **seems unwilling to acknowledge** the restrictions her **increasing** disability will place on her. This **denial may be a coping reaction** to her illness.

- **Presents**: a word redolent of insincerity, pretence, false appearance. The reader is immediately alerted to be suspicious of what follows.
- **Very**: probably unnecessary; 'capable and well-organised' suffices.
- **Determined**: can convey either unreasonable stubbornness or strong commitment to a course of action, depending on the context.
- **Seems**: as with Mrs Woolgar (1) and Mrs Hemmings (4), allows the writer to convey a fact or impression without evidence or commitment.
- **Unwilling to acknowledge**: conveys lack of insight, though Mrs Wheeler might simply not be ready yet to discuss difficult issues, or she might not wish to do so with this worker, or she might be focused on adopting a positive 'can do' approach to her condition: without further specifics, it's not possible to know, we only have the writer's unsubstantiated interpretation.
- **Increasing**: as with Mrs Hemmings (4), instantly indicates history, and in context, conveys failure to be realistic, failure of insight by Mrs Wheeler.
- **Denial**: has a technical function in psychology, and along with diagnoses of medical conditions, provides credibility to the writer, despite the lack of back-up evidence. Reinforces 'unwilling to acknowledge' through repetition of the idea.
- **May be**: like 'seems' above, lets the writer insert the idea into the reader's mind without having to commit themself to the claim – the writer again has a let out.
- **Coping reaction**: as with 'denial', the writer has used semi-technical language and thereby gained otherwise unearned credibility.

General points

1. The emboldened words convey strong pictures and impressions, without sufficient evidence or measured qualification.
2. Without context or evidence, descriptions are received by individual readers and listeners in widely differing ways, as each has their own context from which to fill in the gaps.
3. Each person is described in the third person, without being quoted directly themselves.
4. The scenarios suggest no engagement with the people they describe.

The writer has all the power, the person they write about has no opportunity to intervene in what has been written about them.

Knowing what to include and how to put it

Social care staff expect to record details about service users and their work with them, but it's not always clear or straightforward why they record the information they do, and for whom they are recording. Assessment should involve service users as active partners.[7] 'Person centred planning is a process for continual listening and learning, focusing on what is important to someone now and in the future, and acting upon this in alliance with their family and friends.'[8]

---

[7] Department of Health: Fair access to care services: guidance on eligibility criteria for adult social care, §28 and 35.
[8] Department of Health: Valuing People: a new strategy for learning disability for the 21st century, Ch2 Definition.

✓ Exercise 15: For whom are we recording and for what purpose?

↗ Objective

To assess how clear participants are about why they record and for whom

⏱ Timing

Allow 30 minutes for this exercise.

✎ Materials

- HO 5: Transcript for Vincent Morris (Chapter 1)
- HO 26: For whom are we recording and for what purpose?
- HO 27: Tools to help conduct and record good assessments
- HO 28: Personal Checklist: For whom are we recording and for what purpose?
- Pens
- Flipchart paper and marker pens

ⓘ Trainer's guidelines

Step 1: allow 15 minutes
Divide participants into pairs, each either A or B. With an odd number, make one group three, with the third acting as an observer. Give out HO 5 and ask them:

1. To read the transcript (5 minutes).
2. A to role play Vincent, B to role play Lucy (10 minutes).

Step 2: allow 15 minutes
Bring participants back to the full group to share the key points they listed in their role play.

Step 3
Give out HO 27: Tools to help conduct and record good assessments and HO 28: Personal Checklist: For whom are we recording and for what purpose?

📄 HO 26: For whom are we recording and for what purpose?

1. Read the transcript of Lucy's and Vincent's previous contact (5 minutes).
2. A will role play Vincent, B will role play Lucy (10 minutes).
3. B will make notes of how to record these aspects of Vincent's assessment.
4. Return to the full group to share the points you agreed for Vincent's assessment.

Scenario: Vincent Morris (first encountered in Chapter 1)

Lucy has to write her assessment of Vincent's needs after her visit, and as Vincent has always shared his assessments with Nicholas, she contacts Vincent to discuss what she needs to write before completing the agreed copy.

Considerations

1. Vincent needs appropriate services while Nicholas is away.
2. Vincent is reluctant to let Nicholas know of his worries about their relationship.
3. Lucy is mindful of her duty of confidence to Vincent.
4. Her assessment needs to obtain for Vincent the most appropriate help and support.

It's all in the Record

Trainer notes

1. Vincent needs appropriate services while Nicholas is away:

- Managers making resource decisions need all information relevant to his assessment.
- Service providers need information relevant to his needs, and how they will meet them.
- Workers supporting Vincent need to know any contingency arrangements.
- Workers need to know of any risks they might need to manage.

2. Vincent is reluctant to let Nicholas know of his worries about their relationship:

- Lucy can't force Vincent to share his worries with Nicholas. She can, however, help him work out the pros and cons of sharing or not sharing them.
- Cons include: the risk of exposing how shaky the relationship is; of triggering its end.
- Pros include: the stress of continuing uncertainty doesn't support optimum health and well-being; Nicholas might currently misunderstand Vincent's mood and preoccupations and himself have fears that sharing could resolve; if their relationship is as shaky as Vincent fears, some other factor he can't control could trigger its ending.

This could enable Vincent either to share his fears with Nicholas, or if not, to plan contingencies with Lucy if his fears are realised. If he feels unable to do either, then Lucy might be clearer as to any concerns about his state of mind.

3. Lucy is mindful of her duty of confidence to Vincent:

- Lucy isn't an independent agent, she works for the agency responsible for Vincent's service provision, so she needs to be clear with Vincent that when he confides in her, his information is shared on a need-to-know basis only, within her agency.
- The agency, represented by Lucy, owes Vincent a duty of confidence. She can only share his information with others outside the agency with his consent or if there are pressing reasons to override it. Unless Vincent agrees to letting Nicholas know the fears he's confided in Lucy, she can't let Nicholas have the information.

4. Her assessment needs to obtain for Vincent the most appropriate help and support:

- With Vincent's participation, she can write an assessment that covers everything he's comfortable to share with Nicholas.

She can do a risk assessment[9] based on what could happen if Vincent's fears are realised, as far as possible, with his participation. This would be given on a need to know basis to, for example Vincent's GP, on Vincent's case record in Lucy's office, key service providers: those Lucy and Vincent agree need to be able to respond to an emergency.

---

[9] See Risk assessment in relation to recording and sharing information, HO 31.

HO 27: Tools to help conduct and record good assessments

Best practice is based on key principles of partnership, openness and accuracy. Effective recording is part of the total service to the user. Social service departments need to give clear guidance and training which promotes working in partnership with service users and carers. This includes constructing and sharing written records.[10]

- See service users and carers separately to discuss their own individual needs. This might require using other means than written English.
- Seeing people separately can help check if they really have expressed their own views and wishes, not just what those around them have said.
- Encourage people where possible to write about their needs and circumstances themselves, and complete a self-assessment. This can be a good opportunity to check if your view and theirs agree. Include their own words in your records and assessments.
- Carers and service users do disagree at times. Your assessment risks being ineffectual if you leave out something one has told you in confidence that concerns the other. Show them the result of leaving that key information out. Negotiate with, and enable them as far as possible to express their wishes and views constructively, directly to each other. This can be an opportunity for improved communication, and will free your assessment-writing from being gagged by 'secrets'.
- Write your assessments with people's individual needs and circumstances in mind.
- If people have difficulty expressing their own views, ensure they have access to advocates to help them do so independently.
- Imagine this process of information gathering, concluding things from it, and passing the information and conclusions on to others was about you or a close relative: how would you have felt? How would you have wanted your information to be handled? That consideration is an abiding yardstick for how to record and share personal information.

Including other people's views

- Don't rewrite other people's views so that it's unclear that they are not your own. Quote them directly, attribute clearly, or attach separately.
- Don't reinterpret the views of others: if you need to précis what they said, check that you accurately reflected their views.
- Where opinions differ (e.g. you, the service user and carer might see risk differently), record those differences.
- If you feel that how others expressed their views isn't very helpful, negotiate constructive alternatives.

Expressing difficult issues

- Expressing opinion is a central part of assessment; dealing sometimes with awkward facts. But make sure you base your opinion on sound evidence, not

---

[10] Department of Health: Data Protection Act 1998, Guidance to social services, S3.2.

on personal values, assumption or speculation. The key check is: do you feel OK about sharing what you've written with the person it's about?

- Be open about important issues (who decides what these are?) there should be no secrecy other than for reasons of legitimate confidentiality, but use language that is sensitive and respectful to those concerned. Ask people you're writing about how they would like it phrased – negotiating language to use can: improve communication and understanding; check that people do understand what you're doing and why; and correct inaccuracies. It empowers people. Their words might be better than yours: ask them if they wish to write any part of it.
- But be ready to write what you assess as important even if the service user or carer might not agree: in which case, record their disagreement alongside your assessment.
- If someone is reluctant for you to include something, what difference will leaving it out make to your recording? Is it significant? If so, maybe its importance wasn't sufficiently clear to the person. Can you explain it differently?
- The service user might be embarrassed about some part of their personal life being recorded. Is it essential to write it? Why, for whose benefit? Can you agree a form of wording they are comfortable with? Is there any reason why the service user themself can't just verbally tell those who need to know?
- What has been left out? Only details that are really confidential, or were some difficult to deal with? To whom and why? Are those gaps making the record less relevant? Is further work or discussion needed to be able to address them in the record?

Quality check after assessment

- Did the service user and carer feel they were actively involved, rather than feel they had been passively assessed – or judged – by you?
- Do they recognise themselves in your assessment, with no surprises?
- Are they comfortable with how you expressed the sensitive issues?
- Do they acknowledge that you expressed differences fairly?
- Do they understand and accept why everything you included is there?
- Are they comfortable about who will get a copy of their assessment?
- Did you manage to cover all relevant issues, including those that seemed 'taboo'?
- Do they feel you included everything that is important, to help make 'the best case' with their assessment?

HO 28: Personal checklist: For whom are we recording and for what purpose?

Some social care workers feel that they are expected to know why they record, and what they should record, without that actually being made explicit. This checklist suggests how social care workers who don't feel entirely confident about this could fill in the gaps:

Personal checklist

1. Do you always feel clear about why you record?

2. Are you always clear about who you're recording for? Does it seem as if you have several readerships?

3. Do you feel clear about what's relevant and not relevant to record? How do you decide? Who helps you decide?

4. Do you always tell people that we keep records about their circumstances, needs, services, and why? Are there leaflets to explain this?

5. Do you share people's records with them? Some or all of the records? Some or all of the people? Routinely or at certain times? Do you know what people's rights are about their records?

6. Are you clear when you shouldn't share information with the service user or others?

If you're not sure of the answers to these questions, your supervisor should be able to help you, either directly or by reference to your agency's induction and training programmes, guidance and procedures, recording and confidentiality/privacy policies.

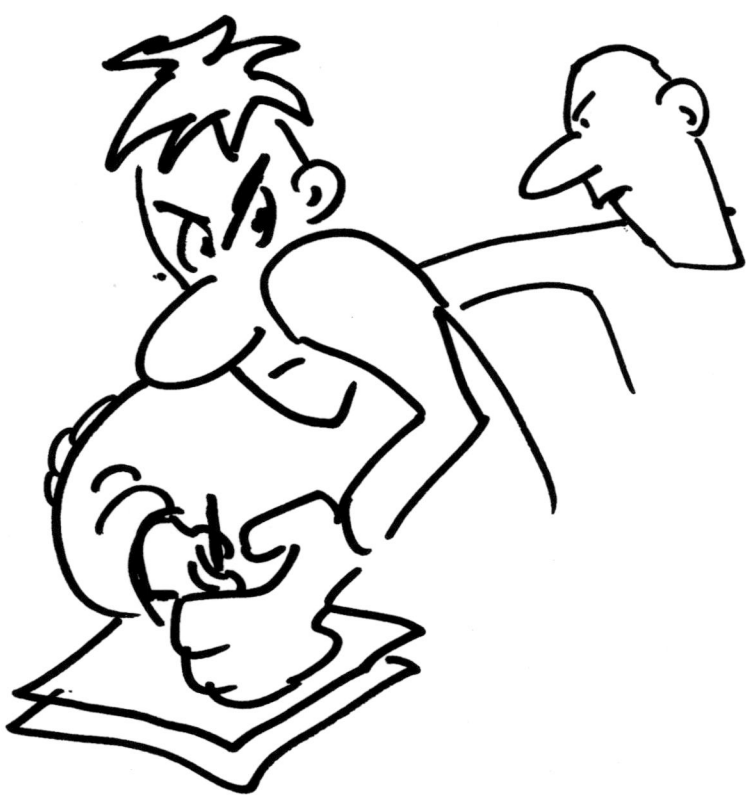

Section C: We know better

We've already explored some circumstances in which personal information can't be shared with the people concerned. But relevant information still needs to be recorded. And it might need to be shared with some, and kept from others.

Usually, records have a 'restricted' section.[11] Care needs to be taken to ensure no more than is necessary is made inaccessible to the people concerned: as we've seen, not sharing information can mean the opportunity to address relevant issues is lost.

Generally, restricted recording is for:

1. Legitimate but speculative information that's not ready to go on the service user's permanent record, nor ready to be shared with others as firm fact or opinion: most likely only shared with the worker's supervisor, to help clarify your thinking or plan next steps to firm up on it. This is the worker's draft, time-limited, thinking-in-progress notes. The worker would expect to transfer this to the permanent, open record when checked out or clearer, or the service user now knows it.
   (Scenarios: Vincent Morris and Jenny Stevenson)

2. Information that a third party requires not to be shared with the person. This might be to protect someone, including the service user, or to avoid undermining the prevention or detection of a crime, which might be against, or by, the service user.
   (Scenarios: Vincent Morris and Mrs Needham)

---

[11] SSI 1997 Inspection Standards on case records, criterion 2.8.

3. Information that the service user indicates they aren't ready yet to deal with, where the information concerns knowledge, insights or understanding that the person isn't ready to hear (for example, someone with a terminal illness), but you need to continue to record the information, and work through it with them when they are ready to do so.
    (Scenario: Bill and Emily Watson)

4. You might use restricted recording in a situation of domestic violence or of a vulnerable adult: to protect the service user from further risk, you might cross-reference the open record to the restricted section, making it clear that this information is not confidential, from the service user, but is not to be given to the relative or person who poses the risk.
    (Scenario: Mrs Needham)

Exercise 16: When recording should be restricted: and to whom or from whom?

↗ Objective

To explore when open recording might validly be restricted: and to whom, or from whom.

🕐 Timing

Allow 60 minutes for this exercise as a whole, or 10–15 minutes per separate scenario, and 15 minutes for a full group round-up.

✏️ Materials

- HO 29: When recording should be restricted: and to whom, or from whom?
- HO 30: Restricting information.
- HO 31: Risk assessment in relation to recording and sharing information.
- Pens
- Flipchart paper and marker pens

ⓘ Trainer's guidelines

Divide participants into groups of four as you give out HO 29: 'When recording should be restricted – and to whom and from whom'. Explain that they will be exploring when it is valid to record information for the use or benefit of some people, while restricting it from others, including the service user.

You may need to note that two of the characters who feature in the scenarios (Vincent Morris in Chapter 1 – Section B, and Chapter 4 – Section B; Jenny Stevenson in Chapter 4 – Section A) have appeared in previous exercises. It is not necessary to refer participants to these earlier exercises in order for them to complete Exercise 16.

Step 1: allow 45 minutes.
Ask participants to decide in each case:

1. What information should be restricted?
2. Who should have the information, and who should not? Why?
3. How might you respond in the light of these restrictions?
4. Should restrictions be permanent, or are there circumstances when they can be lifted? What would they be in each case?

Step 2: allow 15 minutes.
Bring participants back to the full group. Invite them to share what they decided, using the questions above to start the discussion. Note key points on the flipchart.

Step 3
Give out HO 30: Restricting information and HO 31: Risk assessment in relation to recording and sharing information

HO 29: When recording should be restricted: and to whom, or from whom?

Read the following scenarios, and decide (10 minutes per scenario):

1. What information should be restricted?
2. Who should have the information, and who should not? Why?
3. How might you respond in the light of these restrictions?
4. Should restrictions be permanent, or are there circumstances when they can be lifted? What would they be in each case?

Scenario 1: Jenny Stevenson

Jenny is a 23-year-old woman with learning disabilities. She lives in a supported flat. Recently an advocate helped her ask to see her casefile. She wants to know why she left the Lawrences, her foster carers, and went to residential school. Her foster parents stopped fostering after Jenny's placement ended. The records from eight years ago quote the Lawrences as saying that Jenny was sexually provocative and aggressive, and stole money from them. They are also quoted as saying that they felt the social services department gave them very little help at the time. The file doesn't say if any of this was discussed with Jenny, nor whether the Lawrences knew she had a right to see what they said about her.

Scenario 2: Vincent Morris

Vincent is 61, and has lived for 15 years with his 50-year-old partner, Nicholas. Vincent's Motor Neurone Disease was diagnosed five years ago. He uses a wheelchair and has some movement of his arms and hands. He can feed himself but needs help with washing, dressing and using the toilet. Nicholas works full-time for a publishing company as Vincent used to do. Vincent has one home care visit in the morning to help him get up, prepare his breakfast and leave his lunch. Nicholas leaves the house at 6 am and returns at 7 pm, when he prepares Vincent's evening meal and helps him get ready for bed.

Nicholas is going soon to a conference in the USA and then seeing friends. He will be away two weeks in all. Lucy Stratford, social care worker, visits Vincent to assess what he will need during Nicholas' absence, and Vincent tells her that: he's dreading Nicholas going and being on his own for so long; he fears Nicholas leaving him; he doesn't want to talk about it with Nicholas in case he feels more trapped; he feels too dependent on Nicholas for personal care; he has considered suicide if Nicholas left him; there is no-one who could come and stay with him; he no longer sees their friends; he won't consider respite care.

Lucy routinely shares with Vincent the records she writes about his circumstances and needs. Nicholas always opens and deals with Vincent's post and documents.

Scenario 3: Bill and Emily Watson

85-year-old Emily and 83-year-old Bill have been married for 60 years. They ran a shop-cum-post office together, have the same interests, and are very close.

Their family all live some distance away. They have both become quite frail, though still very independent. Bill had a mild stroke a year ago, and now uses a frame to get about. Initially reluctant, they had domiciliary care support since Bill's stroke, and have a good relationship with their carers. Emily fell and fractured her hip 6–7 weeks ago, and has been in hospital since. She has deteriorated quite seriously, developing chest complications and appearing increasingly confused and agitated about where she is and what has happened to her. The doctors agree that she needs nursing care, for some time, if not permanently.

Until last week, volunteers drove Bill to see Emily twice weekly. He spilt boiling water over himself last week while making a cup of tea, and is in a different hospital to Emily for burns treatment. He's very low and distressed at not seeing Emily. His sole concerns are to see her and take her home to be together again. Their family are very worried about how Bill will manage on his own. They are also extremely anxious about how he will take the news about Emily's deteriorating condition, and her not being able to return home as he wishes.

Scenario 4: Mrs Needham

87-year-old Mrs Mollie Needham, a frail, slightly built lady, suffers from severe arthritis in her hands and has had a number of falls. She had a fractured foot a year ago, and had a period in hospital. She can walk slowly and get herself in and out of bed, but needs a commode during the day, and has three visits a week home care support to help prepare meals and help her bathe. Katie Thomas, her home carer, noticed some red marks on her arm. Mrs Needham confided that her son Anthony grabbed her roughly that morning. Katie has been concerned now for some time that Mrs Needham appears to have little in her cupboards and is apparently eating very little. Anthony lives 20 minutes away by car, does the shopping for his mother, cashes her pension, and prepares her other meals. Mrs Needham says he's been drinking, and sometimes gets impatient with her, because she can be so slow, and he has been having money and other worries. His wife left him 3 months ago. She didn't want Katie to do anything, just listen, this is all confidential.

Two weeks later, Katie finds Mrs Needham rather shaky, with a bruise and swelling on her cheek. She denies anything is amiss at first, but when Katie persists, tells her Anthony had been very cross yesterday morning when he called with her shopping as she couldn't find her purse, and he'd pushed her so roughly when he brushed past her at the top of the stairs, that she'd almost tumbled down them. She'd hit her face on the banister.

Trainer notes

Scenario 1: Jenny Stevenson

See Trainer notes on the earlier scenario 3, HO 24. To help decide the appropriate response to Jenny's request, the worker needs to consult the supervisor (and others with expertise if necessary), given such sensitive and unclear information. The worker should identify and record the issues needing clarification. Until they agree on their response, however, recording the detailed considerations (the worker's draft and supervision notes of decisions-in-progress) might need to be restricted: because, if the decision in the end is not to disclose the Lawrences' remarks to Jenny, the information about the process of making that decision could give her some of that restricted information.

- That information would include the assessment of Jenny's ability to handle the information without harm to herself or others.
- If the decision is not to share that information with Jenny, the difficult information should be marked restricted, for future clarity. And whether permanently or otherwise?
- The preferred result will be for the department to share all her information with Jenny, and to offer her all the support she needs to deal with it.
- And to clearly classify the restricted information as part of the open record.

Scenario 2: Vincent Morris

People have a right to privacy: but not to the point where it puts someone at serious risk. Social care workers can't promise confidentiality just between the individual worker and service user. Relevant information is shared in the agency on a strict need-to-know basis.

- Vincent doesn't want Nicholas to know of the feelings he's confided in Lucy. Lucy always shares her records with Vincent. Nicholas always deals with Vincent's papers.
- Lucy is worried about Vincent's fears and talk of suicide. She would like to help him talk to Nicholas, but that is something he needs to decide: he might be right that it would precipitate the thing he fears. He needs to be ready for that risk if he decides to take it.
- Lucy needs to get the right services for Vincent. If her concerns about his mental well-being are well-founded, the services he needs aren't only practical ones. She might assess that he needs counselling and surveillance to minimise the risk of his acting in despair. To obtain those services, she needs to give the reasons to those who agree, and those who provide, the services. She can assure Vincent she won't share his confidences with Nicholas, but her agency needs to know of them.
- Lucy can restrict that part of Vincent's assessment from the copy that Nicholas will see, but will tell relevant managers and service providers. She will identify the information clearly as restricted from Nicholas unless and until Vincent decides otherwise.
- If Vincent decides to share his feelings with Nicholas, then Lucy can move the information from its restricted classification.

- Any restricted information should be reviewed and moved to the open record, when the restriction no longer applies. The desired outcome is for as open a record as possible.

Scenario 3: Bill and Emily Watson

Remember that the law also says that personal information held for social work purposes[12] need not be shared with the person concerned if doing so could cause serious harm to someone: the person concerned or someone else.

- Bill is himself frail and ill, and in need of assessment and services to ensure he can live alone at home safely.
- His whole preoccupation is with returning home with Emily, an aim that the doctors have assessed to be unrealistic.
- Bill is distressed that he hasn't seen Emily since being admitted to hospital himself.

Although it is right to practise open recording, there are times when it can carry risk.

- Bill will have to come to terms with Emily's needs eventually, but those involved in his care will need to plan how to tell him so as not to undermine his own health and well-being. So, the doctors' assessment, and the planning about working with Bill to come to terms with Emily's situation, would be restricted from him until it is judged he is ready to deal with the information without adversely affecting his own health and well-being.
- Meanwhile, if regular visits were arranged for Bill to see Emily now, one of his anxieties would be lifted. He would feel listened to and be reassured in seeing Emily. In seeing her regularly, there is the chance that he might himself come to terms with her condition at a pace he can manage, and so indicate to those working with him and his wife when he is ready to discuss next steps, so the question of restricting information could even be avoided, by meeting another short-term, but equally important need.

Scenario 4: Mrs Needham

Staff should follow their agency's vulnerable adults procedures. Recording should not expose the service user to increased or continuing risk, but at the same time it should inform all who need to know about what has happened, and how it will be managed.

- Katie would not record Mrs Needham's confidences about Anthony's behaviour in Mrs Needham's home-held records, since Anthony could read them and this could increase the risk to Mrs Needham. The risk to Mrs Needham is apparently increasing and Anthony's behaviour is becoming more aggressive.
- Katie can't keep Mrs Needham's confidences to herself, she must tell her line manager. Katie needs to reassure Mrs Needham that, although she must tell her manager, her agency will respect her confidences. If Katie finds Mrs Needham too distressed even for that, then she should not tell her at this

---

[12] The Data Protection (Subject Access Modification) (Social Work) Order 2000.

point, she should avoid adding further to her distress. Katie should record all this carefully for the office-held record. Mrs Needham would have to be told that Katie had acted, but at a later time when it would not adversely affect her health and well-being. The office-held record should explain that Anthony has not been told and also explain whether Mrs Needham knows it is being taken further.

- It is even possible that Mrs Needham confided in Katie because she does in fact want her to act to protect her, but finds it too painful to take responsibility for the consequences. She might hope for the least intrusive action that will both protect her and help rather than punish her son.
- Katie's line manager needs to decide whether to invoke the agency's vulnerable adult procedures. As part of a risk assessment and protection plan,[13] the department might consider e.g. increasing home care involvement to relieve Anthony of the things he does for his mother, and at the same time monitoring the situation more closely.
- The department would normally share her risk assessment and protection plan with Mrs Needham. If the proposed action seemed helpful to both herself and Anthony, it would be unlikely to distress her unduly; though the record might need to be marked as restricted from Anthony, and kept elsewhere than in Mrs Needham's home. If, however, knowing about the department's actions and plans could cause her considerable distress, then they might have to be marked restricted from Mrs Needham also, at least for the time being.
- Restricting information from Mrs Needham and Anthony is not necessarily a permanent condition. Once risk has passed, 'de-restricting' information should be considered. It is possible that, given in the right circumstances, it would benefit Mrs Needham and Anthony if he was told. He too has rights in relation to information about him, though not at the expense of his mother's health and well-being.

A balance needs to be struck between protecting the vulnerable adult, and open recording practices. Protection from serious risk comes first, but restricted information can and should be 'de-restricted' when the risk it concerns has been dealt with or has passed. In restricting it from some people (in this case the victim and the abuser), however, it is important to ensure that those responsible for dealing with the risk have the information.

---

[13] See Risk assessment in relation to recording and sharing information, HO 31.

HO 30: Restricting information

Scenario 1: Jenny Stevenson

- People are entitled to the information about themselves provided by foster carers, like other social care workers, unless there are exceptional reasons, such as the likelihood of harm to someone, including the person it's about.
- A balance is needed between: people's rights to information about them-selves; and the risk of harm to themselves or others if the information distressed or angered them. You can carry out a risk assessment[14] about what to do with information: what are the risks, and for whom, of telling the service user, or not telling the service user? And of telling, or not telling, others who have a role or responsibility in relation to the service user?
- A department can't withhold people's information from them just because it might cause difficulties for the department, but only if there is risk of harm to someone, or if giving it would interfere with the detection or prevention of crime.
- It may be appropriate not to include your draft recording[15] in the open case record, if your information is speculative, sensitive or unclear, and you need to take advice first from your supervisor, to clarify your thinking or plan how to firm up on it. This is your draft, time-limited, thinking-in-progress notes. You would transfer it to the permanent, open record when checked out. If the information indicates risk to someone, you should seek immediate advice about whether you should record it and how.

Scenario 2: Vincent Morris

- People have a right to privacy: but not so it puts someone at serious risk.
- Social care workers can't promise confidentiality as a matter just between the individual worker and the service user. Relevant information is shared within the agency on a strict need-to-know basis.
- Information might be restricted *from* a person(s), or *to* a person(s).
- Any restricted information should be reviewed and moved to the open record, when the restriction no longer applies. The desired outcome is for as open a record as possible.

Scenario 3: Bill and Emily Watson

- The law says that personal information held for social work purposes[16] need not be shared with the person concerned if doing so could cause serious harm to someone: the person concerned or someone else.
- It is justifiable not to share information with someone who indicates they aren't ready yet to deal with it, where it concerns knowledge, insights or understanding that they aren't ready to hear (e.g. someone with a terminal illness), but you need to continue to record the information, and work through it with them when they are ready to do so.

---

[14] See Risk assessment in relation to recording and sharing information, HO 31.
[15] See General on next page.
[16] The Data Protection (Subject Access Modification) (Social Work) Order 2000.

- Meeting one need can help overcome the block on dealing with others. Feeling that you have been listened to can enable someone to listen to what others need to say.

Scenario 4: Mrs Needham

- You might use restricted recording in a situation of domestic violence or of a vulnerable adult: to protect the service user from further risk, making clear this information is confidential, not from the service user, but from the person who poses the risk.
- You should follow your agency's vulnerable adult procedures. Recording should not expose the service user to increased or continuing risk, but at the same time it should inform all who need to know about what has happened, and how it will be managed.
- You should tell people what you are going to record, and what you will do with the information, unless you have reason to believe that telling them will itself be harmful. You should tell them, though, once the risk of harm is past.
- Record restrictions on information clearly, so it is evident who knows, who should not know, why, and when the restrictions no longer apply.
- People can tell you things in confidence, wanting you to act, but fearful of taking responsibility for any action you take, or wanting to minimise the consequences.
- Restricting information is not necessarily a permanent condition. Once risk has passed, 'de-restricting' information should be considered. Being open where possible can help people address their real problems, and respects their rights.
- Strike a balance between protecting a vulnerable adult, and open recording practices. Protection from serious risk comes first, but restricted information can and should be 'de-restricted' when the risk it concerns has been dealt with or is past. In restricting it from some people (in the case of a victim and an abuser), however, it is important to ensure those responsible for dealing with the risk have the information.

General points

- 'Draft' recording: exactly what information is 'draft', and how to deal with it, will usually be covered in agencies' case recording policies and guidance, with set timescales for writing up records. It may differ between authorities and agencies, and will depend on the type of system in general use: paper files or electronic records. It's easier to see your 'work-in-progress' notes tucked briefly into the front of a paper file pending confirmation, than into a more formal electronic record which gives wider access. With the advent of the eSCR (electronic Social Care Record), recording will move wholly to electronic records. Generally, 'draft' information will be short-lived and within a short period either be destroyed as being irrelevant, or firmed up into formal records. Its inclusion and accessibility should be based on the purpose of recording it in its current state, and what are the consequences and risks in recording it or not, and by when. Information that proves unreliable will need to have corrections notified to recipients.
- Restricted information should be clearly marked or classified as such. It should be safe to infer from records that information that isn't restricted forms part of the open record.
- Restricted information isn't always permanently restricted. It should be reviewed on a consistent basis, and moved to the open record when restriction is no longer justified.
- In general, third parties should be encouraged to allow their information to go on the open record, unless it is clearly inappropriate to do so.
- The less that information is restricted, the easier it is to work with people: there are no 'no go' areas in problem-solving and meeting needs.
- Restricting information is appropriate and necessary when it is to protect people.

▣ HO 31: Risk assessment in relation to recording and sharing information

Just as you carry out risk assessment in relation to service users' social care needs, risk assessment is valid for what to do with difficult information. Staff use a range of risk assessment tools, but in relation to recording and sharing information, the key considerations are the same. They include the following:

- For whom is the information difficult? And why?
- Risks to an individual need to be weighed against those faced by carers, family and the wider community, in order to reach a balanced judgement.
- It's important to measure the impact of taking, or not taking, certain actions and decisions – on the service user, carers and community. Identify the risks – and to whom – of giving, or not giving, the information to the service user, their carers and immediate family, the agencies meeting their needs, or others responsible for their safety and well-being.
- When someone is determined on a given course, which those working with them can't support, there are two main considerations:
  1. The safety or well-being of the person and others: are they sufficiently in doubt, or the risk to them substantial enough, to justify action counter to their wishes?
  2. Has the person demonstrated a sufficient awareness of all the risks involved, and the implications of living with them?
- The only person who can consent to the use of personal information is the person it's about. But if they lack insight, risks will be more apparent to others than to them. If someone has been assessed as lacking mental capacity, you might need to decide what to record and what to do with the information on their behalf: in consultation with appropriate professional and family carers (provided there is no conflict of interests) to agree what is in their best interests.
- But people can lack capacity at times rather than always; capacity can be limited rather than absent; stress and unfamiliarity can impair capacity. If people have impaired or variable capacity, you should choose the optimum time, situation and communication methods to consult them.

Section D: For all to see

The principles of partnership, openness and accuracy as the basis of best practice involve a particular challenge for home care workers to record each visit and tell the next home carer anything important, leaving the records with the service user, where others can read them. Information might be sensitive, embarrassing or worrying, and home carers not always sure whether to include or omit it.

   We explored vulnerable adult information issues in the previous section (Mrs Needham and Katie Thomas). It is often clearer whether information should be recorded, and who should have it, where there is an issue of risk. There are other circumstances where the information is difficult, but whether and how to record is less clear.

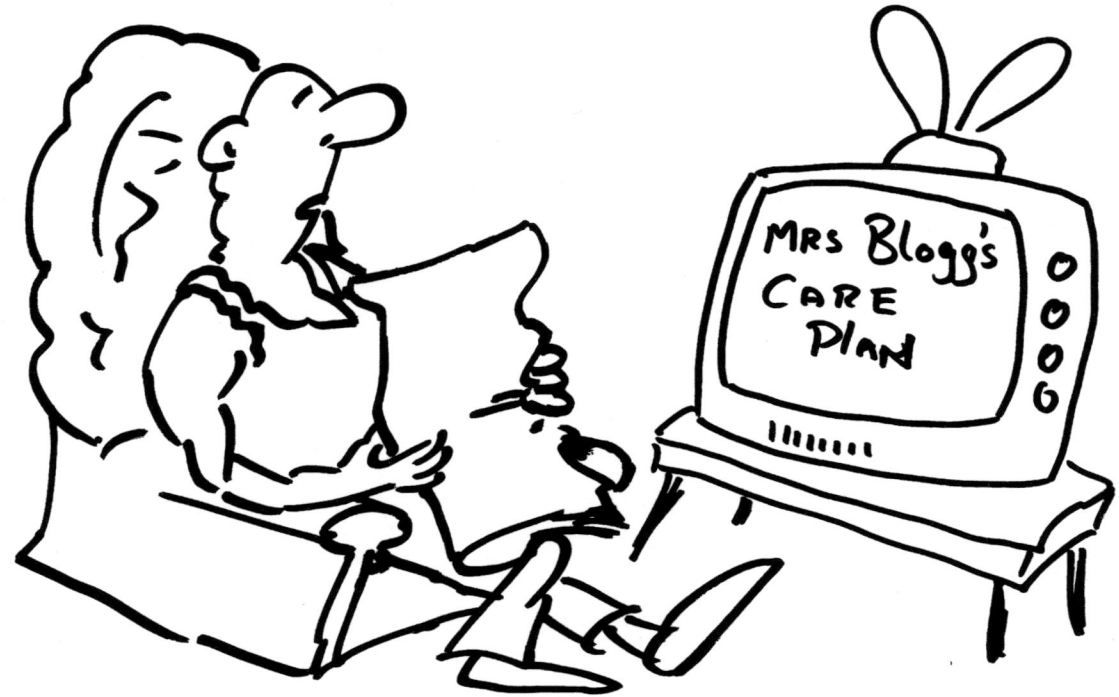

Exercise 17: Information can be embarrassing . . .

↗ Objective

To explore whether and how to record embarrassing (for whom?) information.

🕐 Timing

Allow 45 minutes for this exercise

✐ Materials

- HO 32: Role play: Information is sometimes embarrassing
- HO 33: Issues about the difficulties in recording embarrassing information
- Pens
- Flipchart and marker pens

① Trainer's guidelines

Give out HO 32: Role play: Information is sometimes embarrassing, and explain that participants will be working in groups of four on a four-part role play sequence. Identify each person as A, B, C or D: As will be the service user, Mrs Chester, Bs the home worker, Katie Thomas, Cs the home care supervisor, Nicky Bell and Ds the reviewing officer, Devi Nayar. Participants not making up a complete four will be second Bs (home carer) in groups of five.

Step 1: allow 5 minutes
In the groups of four, participants to read the scenario about Mrs Chester.

Step 2: allow 5 minutes
Role play 1: (A and B) Katie's noticed a smell of urine recently, tries to raise this sensitively with Mrs Chester, and then writes up the record kept in Mrs Chester's home.

Step 3: allow 5 minutes
Role play 2: (B and C) Katie contacts her supervisor Nicky for advice about recording this, and what to do about the recent change in Mrs Chester's personal care and appearance.

Step 4: allow 5 minutes
Role play 3: (C and D) In connection with the forthcoming review, Nicky addresses Katie's concern with Devi.

Step 5: allow 10 minutes
Role play 4: (A, B, C, D) The review is held in Mrs Chester's home. The review addresses Mrs Chester's needs and whether service provision is meeting them.

Step 6: allow 15 minutes
Bring participants back to the full group. Ask the As, then the Bs, the Cs, and the Ds what were the recording issues for them in this scenario. Write these up on the flipchart.

Step 7

Give out HO 33: Issues about the difficulties in recording embarrassing information.

Trainer notes

- See the handout: Issues about the difficulties in recording embarrassing information. It's often more about our embarrassment than of service users'. Avoiding information can mean people's needs aren't most appropriately met.
- Is it ever appropriate not to share information with service users and their families?

Information can legitimately be kept from service users and their families in some specific circumstances, which are explored in the previous and next sections, but as a rule, open recording is the better, more effective option.

HO 32: Role play – Information is sometimes embarrassing

A will role play Mrs Chester, the service user, **B**, Katie Thomas, the home carer, **C**, Nicky Bell, the home care supervisor, **D**, Devi Nayar, the reviewing officer.

1. In fours, read the following scenario (5 minutes).
2. Role play 1: (A and B) Katie's noticed a smell of urine recently, and tries to raise this sensitively with Mrs Chester, then writes up the home-based log (5 minutes).
3. Role play 2: (B and C) Katie contacts her supervisor Nicky for advice about what to record, and what to do about it (5 minutes).
4. Role play 3: (C and D) Nicky contacts Devi about issues relevant for the forthcoming review (5 minutes).
5. Role play 4: (A, B, C, D) The review is held in Mrs Chester's home. Changes are recorded for the review report that every participant will have a copy of (10 minutes).
6. Then rejoin the full group to share your observations about the recording issues (15 minutes).

Scenario 1: Mrs Ellen Chester

Mrs Chester is 89-years-old. She lives alone, having lost her husband 10 years previously. There is no family living nearby, her daughter lives in Australia. She has a respiratory/heart condition and is constantly short of breath. She also has eating difficulties, because of gall bladder problems. Her general health means she can't have an operation for it. So, her chronic nausea and lack of appetite are controlled, not entirely satisfactorily, by medication, but she is underweight and frail in consequence. She finds carrying things, and getting up and downstairs, difficult. The OT assessed her needs a while ago and supplied equipment, which Mrs Chester finds helpful. She also has help with her laundry, essential household tasks and some meal preparation for her special dietary needs.

A few weeks ago, the home carer, Katie Thomas, detected a slight smell of urine in Mrs Chester's home. Mrs Chester and her home have always been pristine till now. Katie asked Mrs Chester whether she was having any new problems she needed help with, but Mrs Chester said not. Over the weeks, Katie has detected an increasingly noticeable smell of urine when near Mrs Chester, and Mrs Chester's clothes looking less clean and neat than previously. Katie told Mrs Chester she was worried that she seemed to be less well than before, but Mrs Chester said she was all right. Katie felt awkward about what to write on the record in Mrs Chester's home, so consulted her supervisor, Nicky Bell, about what to record about the situation, and whether she should tell anyone else.

A review of Mrs Chester's care plan is due in the next month, to be carried out by Devi Nayar, reviewing officer.

HO 33: Issues about the difficulties in recording embarrassing information

To avoid embarrassing Mrs Chester, why record this at all, can't we just tactfully raise it verbally and confidentially with each other on a need-to-know basis? After all, Mrs Chester doesn't seem to be aware of it, or willing to acknowledge it.

- Mrs Chester's health is fragile and this is a change in personal care and appearance. It might be a symptom of deteriorating health which needs attention, so would need to be broached with her, to avoid the risk of failing in our duty of care.
- If you log this only in the office-held record without raising it with Mrs Chester, and refer it confidentially to the District Nurse or GP, this can tie their hands: they won't then be free to be frank with Mrs Chester about the referral, or be able to deal straightforwardly if Mrs Chester's response conflicts with Katie's observations. And what benefit does the information have for Mrs Chester in the office-held record?
- Even if you record this elsewhere or tell each other verbally with the best of intentions, you are breaching Mrs Chester's confidentiality (her consent is required to share it with other agencies), and principles of partnership and openness with service users.
- Mrs Chester also has a right to see her records (the few allowed exceptions don't include information just because it's embarrassing). If information is only verbal, we undermine Mrs Chester's right to know what information we're using about her.
- Keeping information from the person it's about is usually a problem-in-waiting: sooner or later someone forgets, or mentions it, or writes it, so the person finds out about it. The problem is then a much worse one than embarrassment; it's lost trust.
- Perhaps Mrs Chester is too embarrassed to mention it as Katie doesn't. Are they both treating it as too awful to mention? Might not a matter-of-fact observation be better?
- Katie is the worker Mrs Chester knows best, so is the one best able to raise this with her. Katie might need to work out with the help of her supervisor how best to do that.
- Assuming Katie then raises the issue with Mrs Chester, who acknowledges it and agrees to Katie's advice about calling her GP surgery, what should she record? What is the purpose of the home-held log? To log what tasks were carried out and to inform the next home care of relevant issues? Is it necessary to write this in it? For whose benefit? If for Mrs Chester's, Katie could agree the wording with Mrs Chester. Mrs Chester might question why anything needs to be written. That can be a chance for the worker to explain the purpose of the home-held log (perhaps it isn't entirely clear to Mrs Chester), or if unsure, to check with the supervisor if it's OK to leave it out.
- If a worker raises an issue with a service user clearly and respectfully, and the service user denies what is evident, that might indicate that the service user

is unaware. That in turn could suggest confusion or memory loss, which would need appropriate action.

- If the issue isn't confronted when it first becomes apparent, the consequences for effective treatment and care may become worse or more difficult to manage.

Exercise 18: Tricky situation: What should I record?

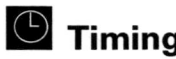 **Objective**

To explore what is relevant information.

Timing

Allow 30 minutes for this exercise

Materials

- HO 34: Tricky situation: What should I record? (Mrs Dexter)
- Paper and pens
- Flipchart paper

Trainer's guidelines

Give out HO 34: Tricky situation: What should I record? (Mrs Dexter) and ask participants to work in pairs.

Step 1: allow 15 minutes
Read the scenario about Mrs Dexter, and decide:

1. What would you record and where?
2. What do you want to happen as a result of the information you recorded?

Step 2: allow 15 minutes
Bring the participants back into the full group to share the problems they had about recording this visit, and how they overcame the recording problems.

HO 34: Tricky situation: What should I record?

Read the scenario (5 minutes), then decide:

1. What would you record and where?
2. What do you want to happen as a result of the information you recorded?

Mrs Dexter is 79 and lives alone. She has no family in the area. She has been receiving home care for the last 18 months, following a diagnosis of Alzheimer's Disease. She is quite clear that she wants to remain in her own home. Home care support involves personal care and meal preparation. Mrs Dexter has no problems with mobility.

This January morning Katie Thomas, the home carer, arrives and finds Mrs Dexter rummaging through her bureau, wearing just vest and knickers. She says she has lost her purse and is sure the neighbour has stolen it. Katie tries to reassure her that she has probably just lost it. Mrs Dexter continues to search for her purse. Katie tells her she really should put some clothes on as it is quite cold. Mrs Dexter has no central heating. Mrs Dexter agrees to go upstairs with Katie but chooses a summer dress. Katie tries to persuade her to put on a jumper or cardigan as well, but Mrs Dexter refuses, saying she is too hot. Katie notices that Mrs Dexter's face is a little flushed. Mrs Dexter continues to complain about the neighbour taking her purse.

Katie asks Mrs Dexter what she would like for breakfast. Mrs Dexter says she would like bacon and eggs. Katie reminds her that there is no bacon. (Mrs Dexter put the last of the bacon in the bin yesterday, saying she didn't want it). Katie offers to cook some eggs. Mrs Dexter is sure she had some bacon and says Katie must have lost it. As Katie prepares breakfast, Mrs Dexter continues to look for the bacon. Mrs Dexter stops in front of the kitchen sink, looking through the window at her garden. She says she knows the neighbour is hiding out there. Katie persuades her to sit down and have breakfast. Mrs Dexter eats half of it, then opens the kitchen door and starts shouting toward the neighbour's house. 'I know what you're up to, I know your game. You've stolen my purse, you buggers'. The neighbour shouts back, 'Shut up you silly old bag or I'll really give you something to complain about'. Katie encourages Mrs Dexter to return to her breakfast, but Mrs Dexter becomes more angry and pushes the plate on to the floor. She goes into her living room and continues to search the bureau.

There is a knock on the door. The neighbour appears and says that he is fed up with Mrs Dexter, calling her 'a batty old cow'. He works night shift and he can't get any sleep with her 'ranting over the fence all the time'. He tells Katie to 'sort her out or he will'. He then returns to his own house. Mrs Dexter comes to the door as he leaves and shouts 'Thief, thief, you've stolen my purse!' Katie persuades her to return indoors. Mrs Dexter goes back into the living room to search the bureau once more. Katie clears up the broken plate and spilt breakfast. She tries again to persuade Mrs Dexter to put on a cardigan but Mrs Dexter doesn't respond. Katie says she can't stay any longer, but reminds Mrs Dexter that June Graham, her colleague, will call as usual at lunchtime.

Trainer notes

What Katie records, and where, depends on a number of factors, e.g.:

- How much insight does Mrs Dexter have?
- Is her record kept in Mrs Dexter's home or elsewhere?
- Is the missing purse an isolated incident or is there a history of Mrs Dexter being unable to find her possessions?
- Although people can blame others for taking things that they have misplaced themselves in their confusion or forgetfulness, people can be vulnerable to exploitation by others. Can the possibility that Mrs Dexter's purse has been stolen be ruled out?
- Has the relationship with the neighbour changed, or is today's encounter fairly usual?
- Are Mrs Dexter's behaviour and appearance as usual, or different today?
- What concerns Katie today?
- What does Katie need to pass on to June Graham, her colleague?

The reasons Katie records and shares information are:

- To account for her work with Mrs Dexter.
- To ensure continuity of service with the next carer.
- To alert the next carer to concerns to monitor.
- To refer concerns that might need to be addressed by her agency via her supervisor.

Katie will need to brief June on:

- What she did today e.g. got Mrs Dexter's breakfast, so she has eaten, though didn't finish it; got Mrs Dexter to put on a dress, but not a cardigan. June will understand this concern, given the weather, season and lack of central heating.
- What is needed: e.g. bacon for tomorrow's breakfast; help if possible to find Mrs Dexter's purse.
- Observations she intends to pass on to her supervisor: e.g. Mrs Dexter looking a little flushed today; she thinks the neighbour has taken her purse; the neighbour's remarks to Katie; Mrs Dexter's remarks to the neighbour.

The considerations about Mrs Dexter's information apply in the following exercise.

Home carers obtain a lot of information, both factual and more speculative, in the course of their work with service users.

Exercise 19: What do I do with this information?

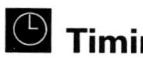 **Objective**

To explore how to choose what is relevant information, and what isn't.

Timing

Allow 30 minutes for this exercise.

Materials

- HO 35: What would you do with this information?
- Paper and pens
- Flipchart paper and flipchart pens

Trainer's guidelines

Depending on the size of the group, divide participants into groups of four, or ask them to work in pairs. Give out HO 35: What would you do with this information? and ask them to read the five short scenarios and decide what they would do with the information. You could suggest some questions for them to start with, e.g: 'What information is important, and why?' 'What would I record, and where?', 'Would I pass any of this on, and if so, to whom, and what would I expect them to do with it?'

Step 1: allow 20 minutes

1. To read the scenarios (5 minutes).
2. To discuss what they would do, as home carers, with this information (15 minutes).

Step 2: allow 10 minutes.
Bring the participants back into the full group to share their decisions. Write key points on the flipchart.

It's all in the Record

 HO 35: What would you do with this information?

1.   Read the scenarios (5 minutes).
2.   Discuss what you would do, as home carers, with this information (15 minutes). What would you record and where? What information would you pass to the office?
3.   Back in the full group, share your views (10 minutes)

1. Mrs Rigby

Mrs Rigby is 81, lives alone and has been diagnosed with Alzheimer's Disease. She does not cook for herself, and because of concerns over her not having an adequate diet, home care now go in once a day in the evening to warm up a meal for her. She does not always like these meals and will sometimes throw them away.

You read in her notes that she ate sandwiches on Wednesday, on Thursday a meal of roast sliced beef was warmed and left for her. You now find most of the remains of that meal in the bin. You ask Mrs Rigby and she says she doesn't like beef any more.

2. Mr Kent

Mr Kent is a 78-eight-year-old man with Parkinson's Disease, who needs help with personal care. He lives with his wife, Kathleen, aged 64. You arrive this morning to find Mr Kent in tears, saying his wife was shouting at him. Kathleen says to you, out of his hearing, that she had lost her temper with her husband. They had never had a very happy marriage, and now she just feels trapped.

3. Mrs Arnold

Mrs Arnold is 85, lives on her own and had a minor stroke three years ago, which affected her left side. She needs personal care and meal preparation. She enjoys listening to the radio, reading the paper and often talks about what is going on in the news.

While talking this morning, she tells you that she thinks the neighbour, who is doing her weekly shopping, is stealing money from her. You ask Mrs Arnold whys she thinks that, and she says that her neighbour is having financial problems. You ask whether Mrs Arnold checks the receipts and change against the cash she gives the neighbour for her shopping. She says she does but the neighbour also buys things from the market and doesn't always get receipts for those items.

4. Mr Pyle

Mr Pyle is 85, lives alone and has been in a wheelchair after being wounded during the Second World War. He tells you he was watching a film on television the previous night and it had upset him. He said that for years he hadn't thought about the war, but in the last few years he had found himself remembering and thinking about many things he wished he'd forgotten.

5. Miss Jackson

Miss Jackson is 67. She was diagnosed with Multiple Sclerosis 20 years ago. She lost her sight 12 years ago and has used a wheelchair for ten years. She lives alone with her cat. The cat is 14 years old has been unwell. It has had at least a dozen accidents in the house in the last month. When you arrive this morning, you find it has messed in the kitchen again. Miss Jackson said she could smell it but couldn't do anything. She said she is feeling unwell, nauseous. She is worried about the cat, saying she doesn't want it put down as it is her only companion.

Trainer notes: Suggested record

1. Mrs Rigby

Contact sheet

Mrs Rigby has not eaten yesterday's meal, found most of it in the bin. She says she does not like beef anymore.

This is important to record as part of the monitoring of Mrs Rigby's food intake in order to ensure she has an adequate diet.

2. Mr Kent

Contact sheet

Mr Kent was tearful on arrival, reported to office.

Passed on to supervisor

Mr Kent was tearful after he said his wife had been shouting at him. Mrs Kent says she lost her temper and that she feels 'trapped'.

This raises difficult issues of how much can be entered in the contact sheets about problems between Mr Kent and his wife. They may find it upsetting to read such details in the contact sheets and may not want such information held in their home. However, it is important to know that Mrs Kent is finding it difficult to cope which may be putting Mr Kent at risk.

3. Mrs Arnold

Contact sheet

Mrs Arnold is worried about an issue which has been reported to the office.

Passed on to supervisor

Mrs Arnold is concerned that her neighbour may be stealing money from her by not giving her the right change when doing her weekly shopping. The neighbour does not always get receipts for items purchased in the market.

It is important to ensure that Mrs Arnold's concerns are not revealed to the neighbour at this point, and so it would not be appropriate to record her suspicions in the contact sheets. However, it would be important to know that Mrs Arnold may be at risk.

4. Mr Pyle

Contact sheet

Mr Pyle said he had been upset by a TV programme which brought back memories of the war.

It is important to record that Mr Pyle has shared his feelings, which might, if they are repeated over time, indicate an area of emotional need with which he might need help.

5. Mrs Jackson

Contact sheet

Mrs Jackson says she feels nauseous. The cat had messed in the kitchen. She is worried about the cat and says she does not want it put down.

Passed on to supervisor

All of the above should be passed on to the supervisor in order to ensure Mrs Jackson is not at risk from infection. However, her feelings in relation to the cat are also important to note.

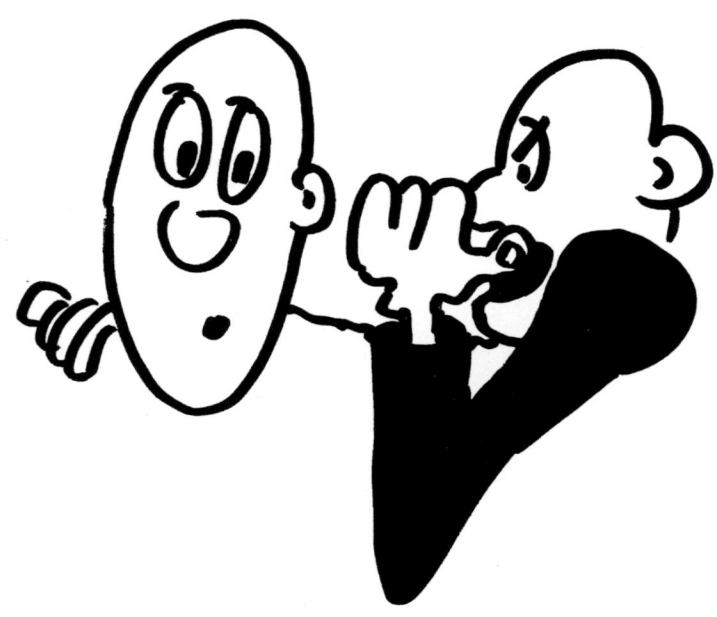

Section E: Have you heard?

Gaining clearance to share information provided by another person with service users in the normal course of day-to-day work is an important way of ensuring that access to records is maximised.[17]

Social services should tell service users why and when information is to be transferred or exchanged between different parts of the service and with provider agencies. They should secure their agreement to this process and ensure that this is clearly recorded. This is an important aspect of people's rights and should mean that, when service users have access to their records, the contents are not a surprise.[18]

Open record policies, which routinely expect all third party information to be shared with service users *unless* confidentiality is specifically stated; together with information-sharing policies, means that sharing information isn't a problem. Staff will be clear when they can and can't share information, and who they can expect to have it.

However, we sometimes need to share information with others about the risks service users face from, or pose to, others. Whereas good practice requires us to routinely gain the service user's consent beforehand to share their information with others, some risks will require us first to consider the impact of doing so: on the service user, on others, and sometimes not seeking consent, or overriding a refusal to give it.

We've already explored third party information, and some of the issues involved in sharing it (or not) in some previous scenarios:

---

[17] Department of Health: Data Protection Act 1998, Guidance to social services, S3.2.
[18] Department of Health: Data Protection Act 1998, Guidance to social services, S3.3.

Third party information: Professional relationships

1. Mrs Margaret Fraser – hospital records (HO 24, scenario 4)
2. Jenny Stevenson – foster carer information (HO 24, scenario 3)
3. Mrs Needham – vulnerable adult issues (HO 29, scenario 4)
4. Bill and Emily Watson – personal expectations in conflict with health assessment (HO 29, scenario 3)

Third party information: Personal relationships

1. Isabel Seymour – individual family member perspectives on the situation (HO 1)
2. Mrs Edith Norman and Mrs Pauline Brent – the clash of individual needs (HO 24, scenario 1)
3. Vincent Morris and Nicholas Baird – the fears about their relationship (HO's 5 and 26)

In the following scenario, we explore the involvement of health and social care workers and the issues around sharing information. This exercise is a useful one for a multi-agency group, for example, those who carry out a single, shared or unified assessment.

Exercise 20: I need to tell someone else

Objective

To explore sharing service users' information with workers from another agency.

Timing

Allow 40 minutes for this exercise

Materials

- HO 36a and 36b (Gerald Harvey)
- Paper and pens
- Flipchart paper and flipchart pens
- HO 36c for the round up/review session at the end

Trainer's guidelines

Explain to participants that they will first discuss in the large group, then work in pairs, then bring back their views on the information sharing issues explored in the scenario. Identify participants as A or B. Give only As HO 36a, and only Bs HO 36b. As will be the district nurse, Bs will be the care manager/social worker.

Step 1: allow 15 minutes
Divide participants into two groups. Tell the first group they are going to take the role of the district nurse in the role play and tell the second group they are going to play the role of the care manager/social worker. Ask them in their groups to think about the issues that they may want to raise in their respective roles and to prepare their negotiating position in the role play.

Step 2: allow 15 minutes.
Ask the groups to now re-form in pairs, with one taking the part of the care manager/social worker, and the other the district nurse. Ask them to negotiate in role a resolution to this situation.

Step 3: allow 10 minutes
Bring the participants back into the full group to share their experiences. Write key points on the flipchart.

What information did the district nurse feel they could share with the care manager/social worker and on what basis? What information did the care manager/social worker feel they could share with the district nurse?

Refer to HO 36c at the end as the standard they'll hear more about, if not already familiar with it, for dealing with personal information.

Scenario

This concerns Gerald Harvey, a 67-year-old man with inoperable stomach cancer.

HO 36a: I need to tell someone else

The district nurse

Gerald Harvey is 67-years-old and was diagnosed three months ago with inoperable stomach cancer. Life expectancy has been put at approximately 12 months. Both he and his wife were told the cancer was inoperable and that chemotherapy would be tried, but neither seemed to want to know any more and did not ask about the future prognosis. Mr Harvey is receiving medication via a pump, which the district nursing team is managing with daily visits. His treatment requires him not to drink alcohol. You are fairly certain there has been a strong smell of alcohol on his breath several times in the last month. When you asked him about it, he denied taking any alcohol. As he is unable to leave the house, you believe that any alcohol he may have drunk has been brought in by his wife. You ask her and she also denies any knowledge of any alcohol. You decide to approach the care manager/social worker, as you feel you have done what you can, and it is up to them to sort out the problem.

In the large group

Identify the issues you are going to raise with the care manager/social worker during your discussion with them.
    Prepare your negotiating position.
    Identify the information sharing issues in this scenario from your perspective.

In pairs

Discuss the situation with the care manager/social worker and try to reach a resolution.

HO 36b: I need to tell someone else

The social worker/care co-ordinator

Gerald Harvey is 67-years-old and was diagnosed three months ago with inoperable stomach cancer. Life expectancy has been put at approximately 12 months. Both he and his wife were told the cancer was inoperable and that chemotherapy would be tried, but neither seemed to want to know anymore and did not ask about the future prognosis. Mr Harvey is receiving medication via a pump, which the district nursing team is managing with daily visits.

The district nurse approaches you, as care co-ordinator, about Mr Gerald Harvey. She explains that she wishes to discuss Mr Harvey with you because she suspects he is drinking alcohol, which is not allowed while he is receiving medication. You are concerned about what the nurse tells you. You are aware that Mrs Harvey is under treatment for depression, but she doesn't want anyone to know that, not even her husband.

In the large group

- Identify the issues you are going to raise with the district nurse during your discussion with them.
- Prepare your negotiating position.
- Identify the information sharing issues in this scenario from your perspective.

In pairs

Discuss the situation with the district nurse and try to reach a resolution.

Trainer notes

- To share personal information, we need their consent, unless there is a justification to set it aside: risk of harm to someone (the person concerned or others); crime.
- Information Governance is what health, social care and their allied agencies and authorities will need to apply in the handling of personal information. Its fundamental principles are known as the Caldicott Principles, listed in HO 36c.
- Risk assessment: what could happen if I do, what could happen if I don't, share the information? Is a helpful tool in deciding if it is justified to do so or not.
- Clearly explaining to service users at the outset that we share information with other agencies, and why, the benefits and safeguards to service users and others, makes staff much more confident about when they can and can't share information with other agencies.
- Putting ourselves in the position of the service user or their close relative and thinking: 'How would I feel if they were doing this with my information? How would I want my information handled?', can help clarify how to do what you need as the worker, recording and sharing information effectively, appropriately and respectfully.

People with capacity are entitled to act in a way that carries risk to themselves; but the worker should ensure that their choice is based on having all the necessary information, and exploring its implications fully.

HO 36c: The Caldicott Principles and Information Governance

Caldicott Principles

Justify the purpose

Every proposed use or transfer of information that identifies individuals (personally-identifiable information) should be clearly defined, scrutinised and reviewed by the Caldicott Guardian. Each Health and Social Care authority has a Caldicott Guardian.

1. **Do not use patient-identifiable information unless it is absolutely necessary.**

   It is necessary to use personally-identifiable information for provision of care. In all other circumstances information should be modified so that some or all of those who might see it are not aware of the individual's identity. For example, case discussions for training purposes in a team do not need to identify an actual person.

2. **Use the minimum necessary personally-identifiable information.**

   Where use of personally-identifiable information is considered essential, the least necessary for the purpose should be used. Ask yourself; do you really need to know that information? If not, don't use it. Remember you too are sometimes the person whose information is being used (at your GP surgery, the hospital etc.).

3. **Access to personally-identifiable information should be on a strict need to know basis.**

   Only those individuals who need access to personally-identifiable information should have access to it, and they should only have access to the information items they need to see. Keep information secure so it does not get into the hands of anyone who should not have it, deliberately or accidentally.

4. **Everyone should be aware of their responsibilities.**

   Action should be taken to ensure that everyone handling personally-identifiable information, practitioner or non-practitioner, is aware of their responsibilities and obligations to respect an individual's confidentiality.

5. **Understand and comply with the law.**

   Every use of personally-identifiable information must be lawful. Each agency needs a responsible person to ensure that the agency complies with their legal requirements.

What is Information Governance?[19]

Information Governance covers the following:

- Data Protection Act 1998
- Freedom of Information Act 2000
- Confidentiality codes of practice

---

[19] Department of Health website: Published: 01.05.04; Reference number: HD1
http://www.dh.gov.uk/PolicyAndGuidance/InformationPolicy/InformationForSocialCare/CaldicottArticle/fs/en?CONTENT_ID=4075306&chk=dvqjYH.

- Information Security Management – BS7799
- Records management

It is wider than the Caldicott Principles, and addresses five broad aspects of information processing – how information is Held, Obtained, Recorded, Used and Shared (HORUS). Policies that involve information processing will need to apply Information Governance standards.

Information Governance has four fundamental aims:

- To support the provision of high quality care by promoting the effective and appropriate use of information.
- To encourage responsible staff to work closely together, preventing duplication of effort and enabling more efficient use of resources.
- To develop support arrangements and provide staff with appropriate tools and support to enable them to discharge their responsibilities to consistently high standards.
- To enable organisations to understand their own performance and manage improvement in a systematic and effective way.

Chapter 5: You Can't Please All of the People All of the Time

In this final chapter we want to highlight a number of dilemmas which practitioners may experience in recording. These dilemmas arise from practitioners' perception of the contradictory demands and expectations placed on recording from the different readerships of the record. Practitioners have identified these dilemmas in training sessions and described their feelings of frustrated confusion in trying to reconcile them.

Inconsistent expectations

The dilemmas sometimes arise from the apparently inconsistent expectations of management. These may be part of the fundamental tension between good practice and the pressure on through put, in other words the basic problem of quality versus quantity. If there are a large number of unallocated cases and government targets to meet in terms of the time taken from referral to assessment, not to mention the problem of reimbursements for delayed discharges, then workers are likely to feel under pressure to process the cases as quickly as possible. At the same time they are being reminded of the importance of person centred practice and the need for holistic assessments. Practitioners feel they are being urged to concentrate on only the most essential information in relation to the eligible needs according to one set of guidelines, and then to provide a rounded picture of the person according to another set of guidelines.

This dilemma is addressed in the section 'Stick to the essentials', HO 38.

Competing for scarce resources

Another dilemma centres around the problem of competition for scarce resources. As advocates for their clients, practitioners want to ensure that they get the necessary resources to meet the service user's needs. However, it has been said by practitioners during training from many different authorities, that they feel experience has demonstrated that they weaken their case if they mention in their reports to resource allocation panels, any 'positives' in relation to what the service user is still able to do for themselves. Practitioners believe that they have to describe the service user in the worst possible terms in order to successfully compete for those scarce resources. This then undermines the notion of holistic assessments as well as having a negative effect on the service user's self-image.

This dilemma is addressed in the section 'Painting the worst picture'.

Driven by the system

Practitioners have also described the way in which they feel their recording is increasingly constrained by the recording system, be it paper based or computerised, which they are required to use. Recording practice is seen as an administrative process rather than the exercise of professional skills. They will say that although they feel certain information is important to record, they do not feel the recording system recognises it as relevant, and effectively discourages recording of that information by having no appropriate box or space in which to enter it.

This dilemma is addressed in the section 'Follow the form'.

Advocate or representative

There are also the concerns that some practitioners feel about the consequences of their recording in terms of how it may reflect on their department. Some practitioners are still unclear about whether to record unmet needs and feel that managers are anxious about recording any needs that the department might not be able to meet. This may also extend to practitioners feeling that they are not supposed to make any recommendations in their assessments, as this might commit the department and provide the service user with ammunition, which they could then use against the department, should those recommendations not be followed. This raises an even larger issue about how recording, by providing evidence of a department's handling of a particular case, may subsequently be the basis on which the department is criticised.

These various issues highlight the problems encountered by practitioners in the difficult and complex business of recording. We would like to provide an opportunity for practitioners and managers to explore these issues. An important step is to acknowledge them and then to recognise the need for clear guidance to ensure that workers are not left trying to reconcile these dilemmas, pulled this way and that by what they perceive as contradictory pressures and inconsistent advice.

This dilemma is addressed in the section 'Washing laundry'.

We are using the device of a fictional character called Annie, who works as a care manager and has been qualified for five years. She has worked in a several authorities and still feels confused over what and how she should record. Each dilemma will be highlighted under a different heading. The dilemma will then form the basis on which learners can explore the issues and identify ways in which to help Annie reconcile the dilemma and to feel more confident about her recording.

Exercise 21: Annie's dilemmas

Objective

To explore the dilemmas and tensions in case recording perceived by practitioners and identify strategies for resolving them.

Timing

Allow 1 hour to 1 hour and 10 minutes for each dilemma

Materials

- HO 37: Painting the worst picture
- HO 38: Stick to the essentials
- HO 39: Follow the form
- HO 40: Washing laundry
- Pens and paper
- Flipchart paper

Trainer's guidelines

Step 1: allow 5 minutes
Introduce the exercise and divide into appropriate number of groups for each dilemma:

- 'Painting the worst picture' requires four groups
- 'Stick to the essentials' requires three groups

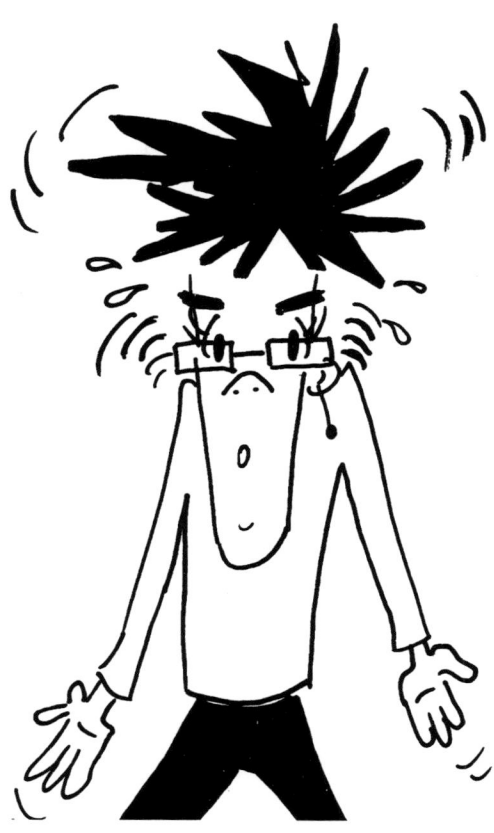

- 'Follow the form' requires two groups
- 'Washing laundry' requires four groups,
- and give participants the appropriate information sheet for the particular dilemma being addressed.

Step 2: allow 20 minutes
Ask participants to discuss the issues from the perspective of their group and prepare to present their position to the other groups, using flipchart paper to summarise their points.

Step 3: allow between 10 and 20 minutes, depending on the number of groups
Ask each group to present their position, allowing approximately 5 minutes for each group.

Step 4: allow 15 minutes
Re-divide the participants into four groups ensuring each group is made up of a mix of representatives from the various previous groups. Ask them to come to a reconciliation of the issue with definitive guidance for Annie and recommendations to management.

Step 5: allow 20 minutes
Each group presents their guidance for Annie and management recommendations using flip-chart paper to summarise their points.

Trainer to review the guidance provided by the groups and refer if necessary to points identified in the Trainer 'points for consideration'.

▣ HO 37: Annie's dilemmas: Painting the worst picture

Annie has been encouraged by her manager to write holistic assessments. Her manager believes it is important to provide information on what the service user can still do for themselves as well as what they cannot do, so that a balanced picture emerges, including strengths and weaknesses. Annie's manager believes this is important in order to arrive at an accurate assessment of the service user's needs, which will assist in making decisions on the most appropriate allocation of resources.

Annie's manager also feels that service providers need to know what a service user is still able to do, so that they do not inadvertently encourage further dependence.

Annie has followed this advice, but is concerned that some of her service users have not always got the resources that she has argued they need. She discusses the problem with a colleague, who seems to be more successful with Resource Allocation Panel reports. Her colleague says that he always emphasises the negatives and plays down the positives. He argues that unless you paint the worst picture your case will not be treated as a priority.

Annie follows this advice, despite her manager's comments about her reports being more negative. Annie finds that her reports are more successful in getting her recommendations approved. Her service users are happy with the outcome, but are quite upset at reading such a negative description of themselves. Some have said that they did not even recognise themselves.

Group A – represents Annie's manager

Group B – represents The Resource Allocation Panel

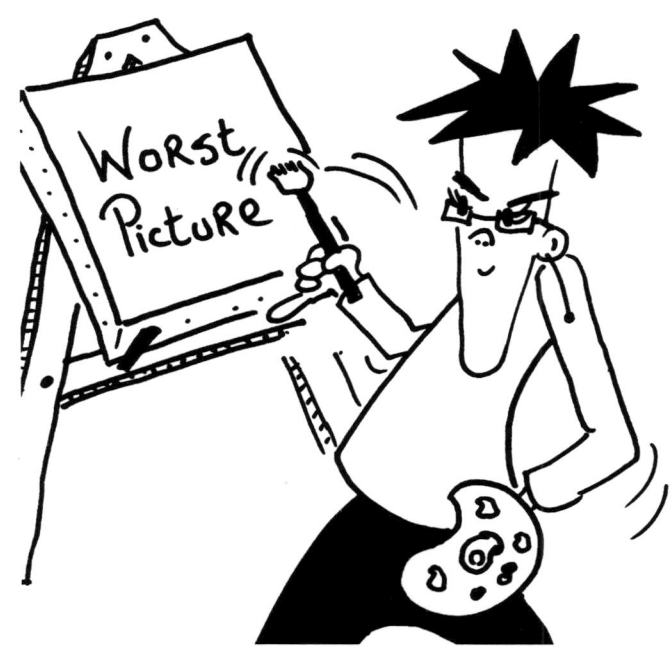

Painting the Worst Picture

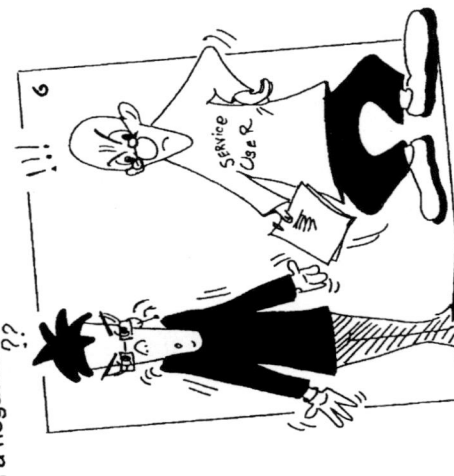

She discusses the problem with a colleague who seems to be more successful with Resource Allocation Panel reports.

Her service users are happy with the outcome but are quite upset at reading such a negative description of themselves.

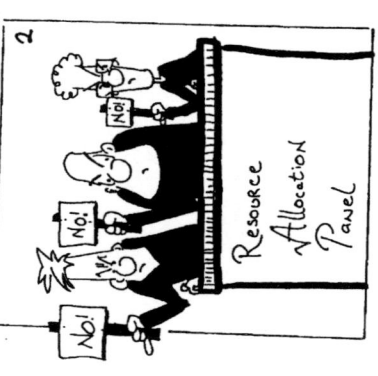

Annie has followed this advice but is concerned that some of her service users have not always got the resources that she has argued they need.

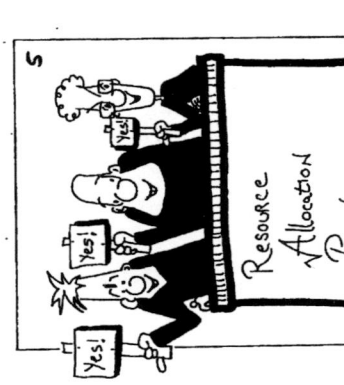

Annie finds that her reports are more successful in getting her recommendations approved.

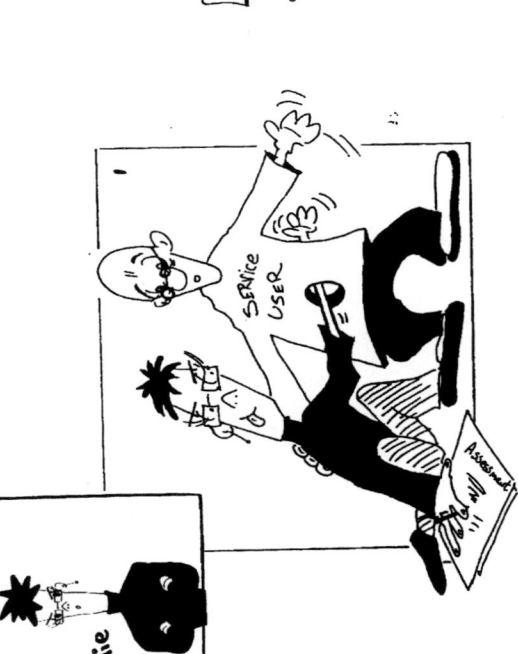

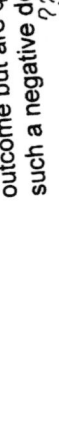

Annie has been encouraged by her manager to write holistic assessments.

Annie re-writes her reports emphasizing the negatives.

Group C – represents Annie's colleague
Group D – represents Annie

Part 1 of exercise

In your first group discuss the issues from the perspective of the person or persons you represent. Prepare to present their position and concerns to the other group/s, using flipchart paper to summarise the points.

Part 2 of exercise

In your reconstituted groups try to reconcile the issues and concerns which have emerged in the previous discussion and provide definitive guidance for Annie and recommendations to management.

HO 38: Annie's dilemmas: Stick to the essentials

Annie finds herself with a new manager, who starts to criticise her recording for being too detailed. Her manager says that she should stick to the point and concentrate only on recording the eligible needs. Annie explains that her previous manager encouraged a holistic, person-centred approach to assessment, one that provided enough background information to understand the service user as an individual. Annie's previous manager felt that you needed to see the person and not the case in the record.

Annie's new manager says that government targets on assessment times mean that she has got to speed up her work, and that she cannot spend so long going into such detailed background information. She should just establish the areas of need against the Fair Access to Care Services criteria, and identify the most appropriate response for meeting those needs.

Group A – represents Annie's new manager
Group B – represents Annie's previous manager
Group C – represents Annie

Part 1 of exercise

In your first group discuss the issues from the perspective of the person or persons you represent. Prepare to present their position and concerns to the other group/s, using flipchart paper to summarise the points.

Part 2 of exercise

In your reconstituted groups try to reconcile the issues and concerns which have emerged in the previous discussion and provide definitive guidance for Annie and recommendations to management.

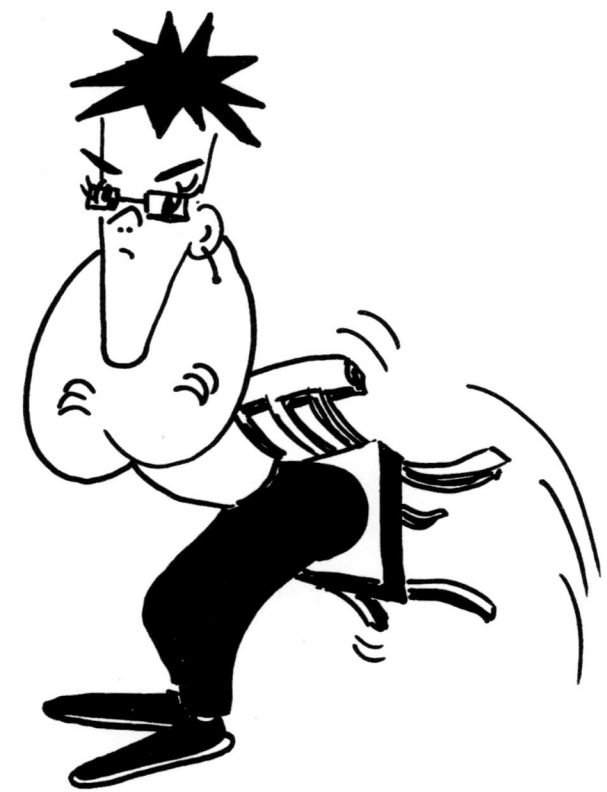

Stick to the Essentials

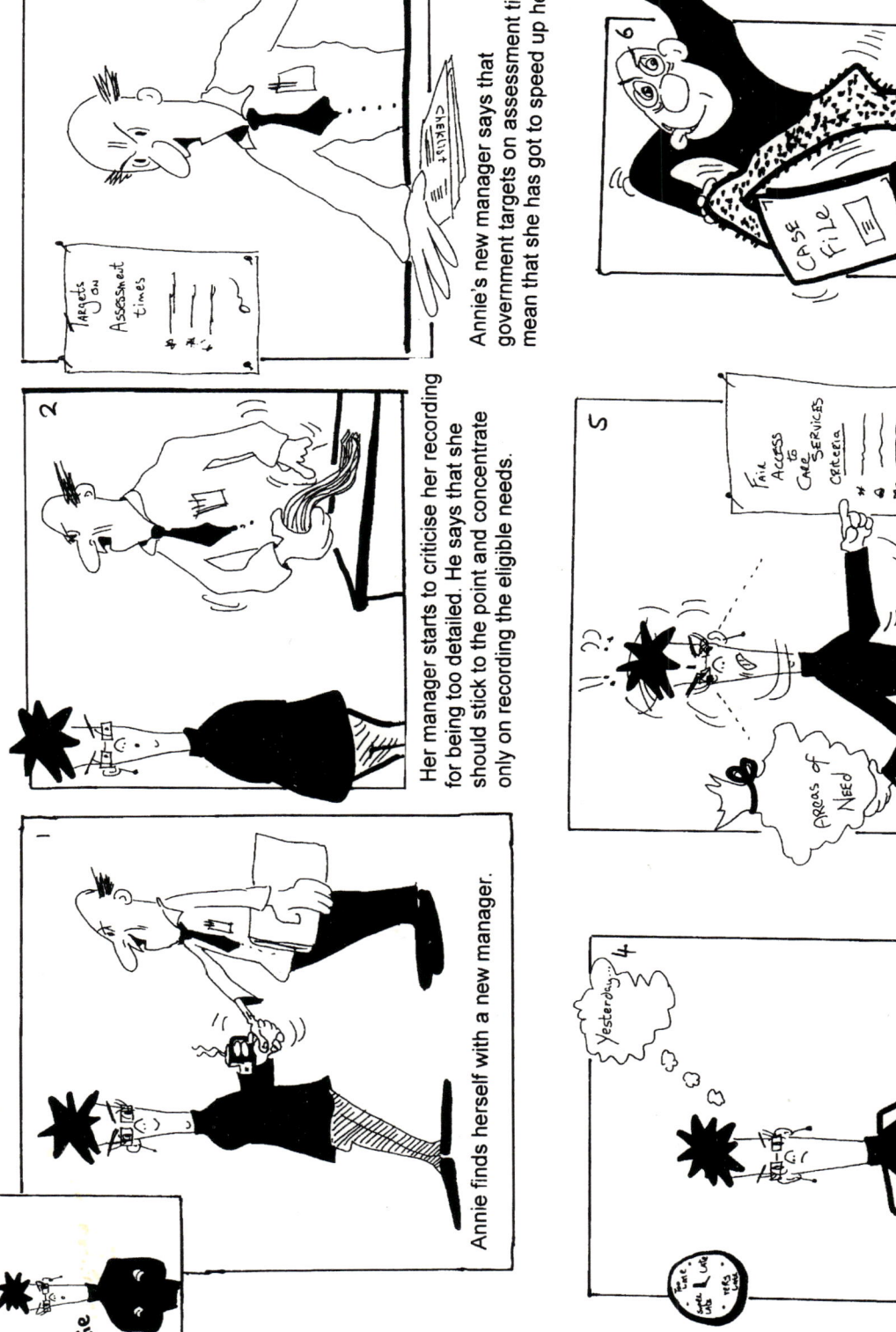

Annie finds herself with a new manager.

Her manager starts to criticise her recording for being too detailed. He says that she should stick to the point and concentrate only on recording the eligible needs.

Annie's new manager says that government targets on assessment times mean that she has got to speed up her work.

She should just establish the areas of need against the Fair Access to Care Services criteria and identify the most appropriate response for meeting those needs.

Annie's previous manager felt that you needed to see the person and not the case in the record

HO 39: Annie's dilemmas: Follow the form

Annie's department has introduced a new computerised record system which she is trying to get used to. Her key board skills are reasonable, better than some of her colleagues, but she finds the new system confusing because she does not know where to record certain information. She has been used to a narrative style of case recording, but has now been told that all her recording should be made under particular headings.

She can see the usefulness of being able to find all the information relevant to a particular area under one heading, but she feels it makes it difficult to see the person as a whole. She is concerned that by recording information under various headings, you sometimes lose a sense of how that information was given by the service user, and how one issue may connect with another, i.e. the way mood and physical health may interact and both be a consequence of the social isolation of the individual.

Annie is also worried that sometimes there does not seem to be a box to record certain information and then she ends up leaving it out, or putting it under a heading that she thinks is vaguely related, but unsure whether other practitioners will see it that way.

Group A – represents those introducing the new computer system

Group B – represents Annie

Part 1 of exercise

In your first group discuss the issues from the perspective of the person or persons you represent. Prepare to present their position and concerns to the other group/s, using flipchart paper to summarise the points.

Part 2 of exercise

In your reconstituted groups try to reconcile the issues and concerns which have emerged in the previous discussion and provide definitive guidance for Annie and recommendations to management.

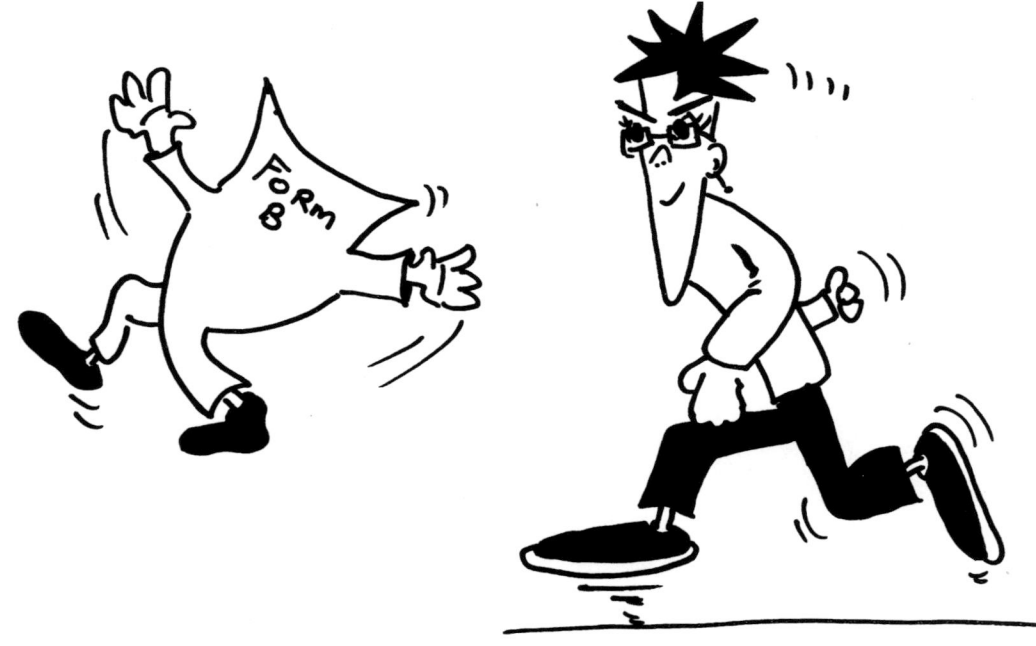

Follow the Form

Annie's department has introduced a new computerised record system which she is trying to get used to.

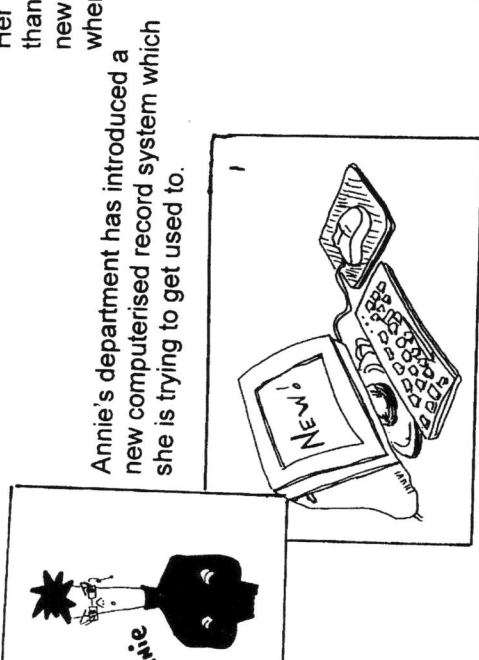

Her key board skills are reasonable, better than some of her colleagues, but she finds the new system confusing because she does not know where to record certain information.

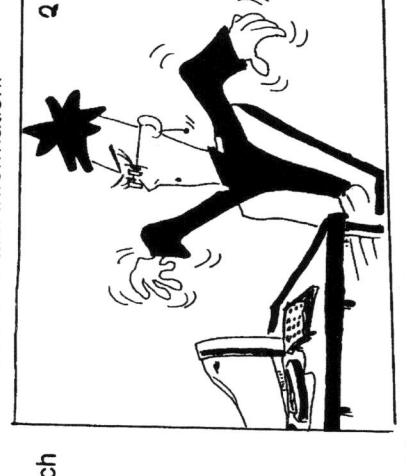

She has been used to a narrative style of case recording, but has now been told that all her recording should be made under particular headings.

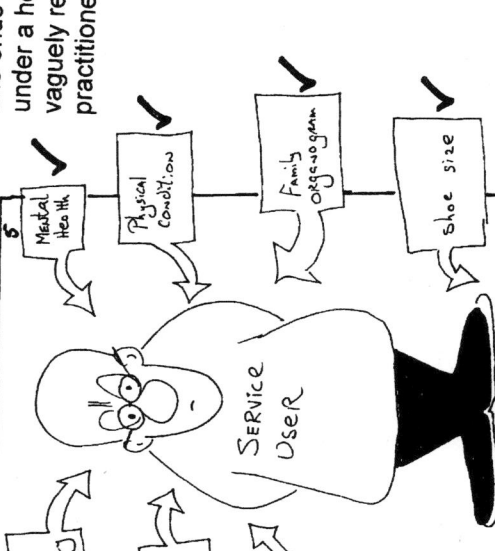

She is concerned that by recording information under various headings, you sometimes lose a sense of how that information was given by the service user and how one issue may connect with another, i.e. the way mood and physical may interact and both be a consequence of the social isolation of the individual.

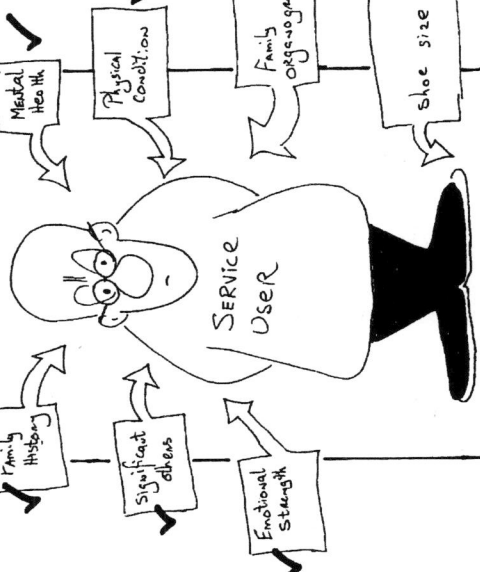

She can see the usefulness of being able to find all the information relevant to a particular area under one heading, but she feels it makes it difficult to see the person as a whole.

Annie is also worried that sometimes there does not seem to be a box to record certain information and then she ends up leaving it out, or putting it under a heading that she thinks is vaguely related but unsure whether other practitioners will see it that way.

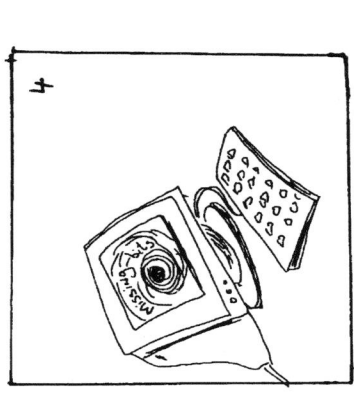

▣ HO 40: Annie's dilemmas: Washing laundry

Annie has found herself in a difficult situation with a service user called Mrs Theresa Thomas. Mrs Thomas, aged 73 was diagnosed with Alzheimer's Disease four years ago. She is cared for by her husband, aged 66, with support from home care.

She has just received a call from the home care supervisor, reporting that the home carers are worried that Mr Thomas is expecting them to dry his wife after washing, using towels which are so rough that they are chafing her skin and causing her distress. The home carers have also complained that the towels are not very clean. When they have tried to discuss the problem with Mr Thomas, he says he has no money for new towels and if they want to buy new ones they can.

Annie visits Mr Thomas. When she calls the home carer is about to leave. She says to you out of Mr Thomas's hearing, that she has been concerned about the problem with the towels for the past three months and kept phoning the office, but no one seemed to do anything. She says she has been really worried about Mrs Thomas and feels that home carers have been asked to go along with cruel and uncaring treatment. She says that she and her colleagues have noted their concerns in the contact sheets kept in the house, but Mr Thomas has become angry and complained to the office. She says that their supervisor advised them to be careful in their recordings and not to upset Mr Thomas.

Annie then speaks to Mr Thomas and explains the home carers' concerns. He restates his position that he has no money for new towels and how do they expect him to manage on the pitiful amount of money he gets. Annie explains that she has explored all the welfare entitlements for both Mr Thomas and his wife in order to maximise their income. Mr Thomas asks her how she would like to live on their income. Mr Thomas says that despite his age he would still be willing to go out and work if someone would look after his wife. He reminds her that he made that suggestion at the time his wife was assessed but was told that would not be possible. Annie recalls that she didn't include it in the written assessment because she believed that there was no possibility of such cover being provided.

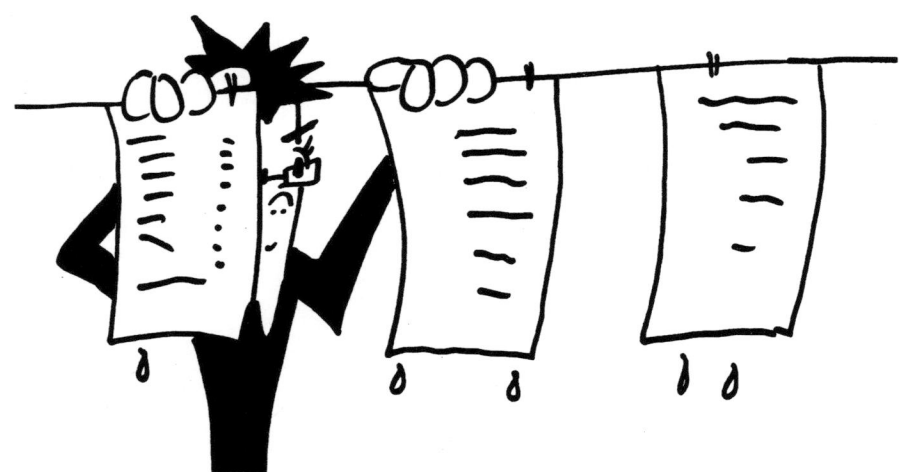

Washing Laundry

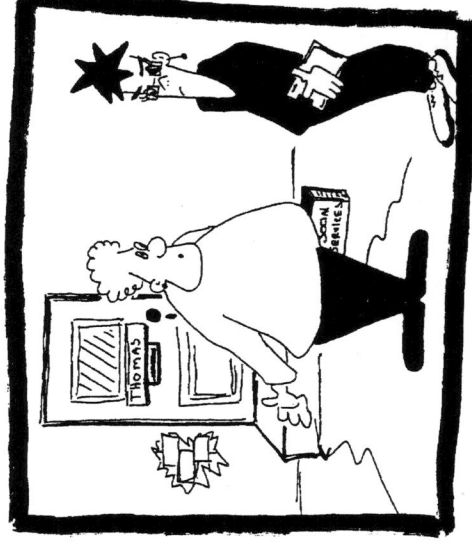

Annie visits Mr Thomas. When she calls the home carer is about to leave. She says to Annie out of Mr Thomas's hearing, that she has been concerned about the problem with the towels for the past three months and kept phoning the office, but no one seemed to do anything.

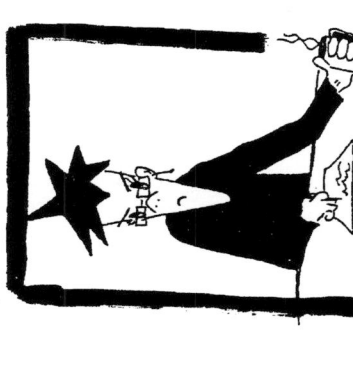

Annie returns to the office with the issue unresolved. Part of her wants to go and buy a set of new towels for Mr Thomas, but she knows that is not the professional response.

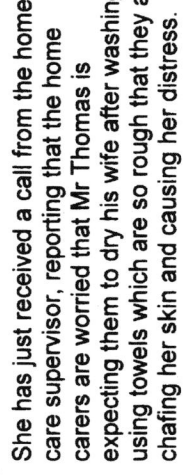

She has just received a call from the home care supervisor, reporting that the home carers are worried that Mr Thomas is expecting them to dry his wife after washing, using towels which are so rough that they are chafing her skin and causing her distress.

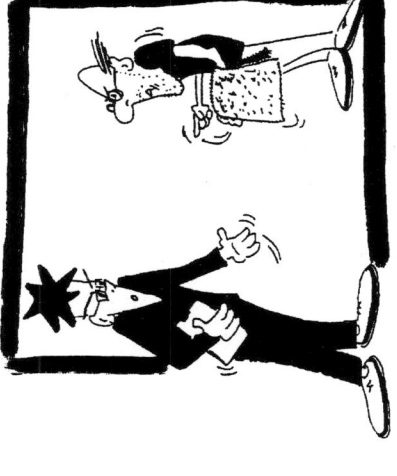

Mr Thomas says that despite his age he would still be willing to go out and work if someone would look after his wife.

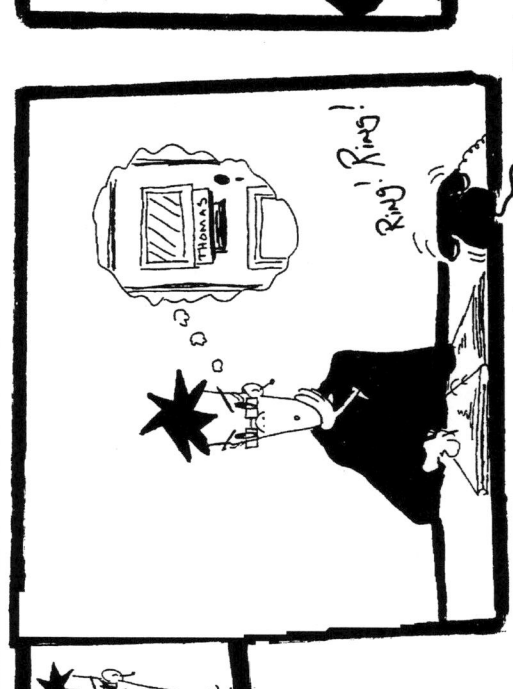

Annie has found herself in a difficult situation with a service user called Mrs Theresa Thomas. Mrs Thomas, aged 73 was diagnosed with Alzheimer's Disease four years ago. She is cared for by her husband, aged 66, with support from home care.

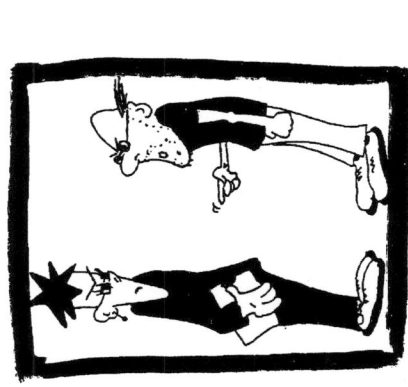

Annie then speaks to Mr Thomas and explains the home carers' concerns.

Annie returns to the office with the issue unresolved. Part of her wants to go and buy a set of new towels for Mr Thomas, but she knows that is not the professional response. At one level the issue seems trivial and at another she knows it is very serious. Mrs Thomas is being caused unnecessary distress for the want of proper towels. She will not be able to talk to her supervisor until the end of the week as she is away on a course. In the meantime she has to decide what to record on Mrs Thomas's case file.

Group A – represents the department's interests
Group B – represents the home carers
Group C – represents Mrs Thomas
Group D – represents Annie

Part 1 of exercise

In your first group, discuss the issues from the perspective of the person or persons you represent. Prepare to present their position and concerns to the other group/s, using flipchart paper to summarise the points.

Part 2 of exercise

In your reconstituted groups try to reconcile the issues and concerns which have emerged in the previous discussion and provide definitive guidance for Annie and recommendations to management.

Points for consideration

Painting the worst picture

1. Do practitioners see themselves as advocates, representing the service user's case to the Resource Allocation Panel or departmental representatives assessing a service user's needs?
2. Does the department explain to practitioners its expectations of their role in the submission of reports to the Resource Allocation Panel?
3. Do Resource Allocation Panels give practitioners detailed feedback on their reports, explaining why a decision was made?
4. Is there a process to monitor the decisions of Resource Allocation Panels?
5. Does the induction of new staff include clear guidance on the criteria used by Resource Allocation Panels in making their decisions?
6. Is there an opportunity for new staff to join a Resource Allocation Panel meeting as an observer?

Stick to the essentials

1. Is there clear guidance to practitioners on the level of detail required in an assessment and is that detail dependent on the size of the care package?
2. Is there guidance and support for practitioners in prioritising work?
3. Is there a regular process of giving feedback to practitioners on the quality of their assessments?
4. Are practitioners able to follow model assessments as practical examples of the level of detail required in a particular level of assessment?
5. Is there a system for ensuring a consistency of standards and expectations of assessments throughout the department?

Follow the form

1. Is training available not only on the lay-out of the form but how to use it, i.e. what information goes where?
2. Are there guidelines on how to record information that does not fit into an obvious category?
3. Is there a process for monitoring the implementation of a new recording system, where feedback can be used to modify the system when necessary?
4. With the introduction of a new form is there a review of existing paperwork to identify whether it has resulted in any unnecessary duplication of information which could be reduced?
5. Are staff encouraged to make suggestions on how recording systems could be improved?

Washing laundry

1. Is there clear guidance on the duty and expectations on staff in respect of recording information, which may expose the department to criticism or liability?

2. Is your department characterised by a blame culture, where problems are always seen as failings of individuals rather than ineffective systems?
3. Are mistakes openly acknowledged and used as opportunities to learn and improve performance both of individuals and the organisation?
4. Is there clear guidance to practitioners on the recording of unmet needs?
5. What lessons would practitioners draw from the way they see complaints dealt with by the department?
6. Is there a clear process for home care workers to add information and concerns to the service user's record?

General points

1. Is there clear guidance to new staff in relation to expected standards of recording practice in the department?
2. Do staff receive regular feedback on their recording practice?
3. Are there opportunities for teams to identify and share good practice in recording and so encourage professional development?
